AF580519

CANCER ETIOLOGY, DIAGNOSIS AND TREATMENTS

OLIGODENDROGLIOMAS (ODS)

DIAGNOSIS, OUTCOMES AND PROGNOSIS

CANCER ETIOLOGY, DIAGNOSIS AND TREATMENTS

Additional books in this series can be found on Nova's website under the Series tab.

Additional e-books in this series can be found on Nova's website under the e-book tab.

CANCER ETIOLOGY, DIAGNOSIS AND TREATMENTS

OLIGODENDROGLIOMAS (ODs)

DIAGNOSIS, OUTCOMES AND PROGNOSIS

CHAD REEVES
EDITOR

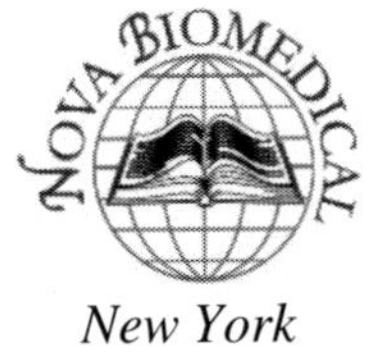

New York

Library of Congress Cataloging-in-Publication Data

LCCN: 2015956842

ISBN: 978-1-63484-278-5

Published by Nova Science Publishers, Inc. † New York

CONTENTS

PREFACE

Cancer is the second leading cause of morbidity and mortality worldwide, ranking just after cardiovascular diseases. In the central nervous system, gliomas constitute the most frequent type of tumors. According to the definition, oligodendrogliomas are diffusely infiltrating glial tumors, composed of neoplastic oligodendroglial cells, typically found in cerebral hemispheres in adult population, although not uncommon in children. They encompass a range of tumours, from well-differentiated to frankly malignant neoplasms. In the current World Health Organization (WHO) classification of tumors of the central nervous system, covering a four-tiered WHO grading scheme, oligodendrogliomas are recognised as grade WHO II and WHO III by the degree of malignancy. They may be either well differentiated, composed of neoplastic cells that morphologically resemble oligodendroglia, or may harbor focal or diffuse features of malignancy, respectively. Their prognosis is in this case less favorable. This book provides current research on the diagnosis, outcomes and prognosis of oligodendrogliomas. Chapter one examines the pathology, molecular mechanisms and clinical references of ODs. Chapter two discusses the ODs and the problematic diagnostic markers. Chapter three examines the histopathologic features of oligodendrogliomas and of an assortment of other central nervous system neoplasms that can resemble them and reviews features that allow one to sort through these histopathologic differential diagnoses. The final chapter reviews speech mapping in oligodendroglioma operations and provides data regarding patient outcomes with these methods.

Chapter 1 – The chapter is based on a personal experience of 253 cases of oligodendroglial gliomas, composed of 122 grade II oligodendrogliomas (OII), 55 grade II oligodendrogliomas (OIII), 51 grade II oligoastrocytomas (OAII),

12 grade III oligoastrocytomas (OAIII) and 13 grade IV glioblastomas (GBM) with oligodendroglioma component (GBMO). Oligodendrogliomas are more frequent in men than in women with a peak incidence of 45 years of age. In recent years, an increased incidence rate has been observed. They appear as well demarcated lesions, hypointense at T1 and hyperintense at T2 magnetic resonance imaging (MRI). Epileptic seizures and focal signs are the main clinical features. According to the World Health Organization (WHO) classification of tumors of the central nervous system (CNS), the following histologic types can be distinguished: OII. Diffuse growth and occurrence of the so-called "honeycomb" appearance and vessels with a "chicken-wire" distribution. Calcifications are frequent. OIII. Vascular proliferation, endothelial hyperplasia and microvessel proliferation. High cell density, high number of mitoses, circumscribed necroses. OAII. Occurrence of both an astrocytic and an oligodendroglial component. The main problem is the distinction of tumor from reactive astrocytes. OAIII. Nuclear atypias, microvascular proliferations (MVPs), circumscribed necroses and high mitotic rate. The real existence of OA as distinct tumor entity is today denied or discussed. GBMO. It is discussed as either glioblastoma of oligodendroglial origin, OIII or as real tumor entity. Immunohistochemistry. It concerns multiple markers such as myelin basic protein (MBP), myelin-associated glycoprotein (MAG), PDGFRα, NG2, CNPase, MAP2, OLIG1 and OLIG2, glial fibrillary acidic protein (GFAP) and the proliferation index Ki-67/MIB-1. Molecular genetics. Of great importance in diagnosis and prognosis, it includes 1p/19q co-deletion, somatic IDH1/2, TERT, CIC, FUBP1, TP53 and ATRX mutations, MGMT and EMP3 hypermethylation, CDKN2A/CDKN2B copy number changes. Prognosis and therapy. The tumors are more benign than the corresponding astrocytic tumors of the same histologic grade. The prognosis depends on the grade of malignancy, histology and the genetic asset. Prognostic markers are the proliferation index Ki-67/MIB-1, 1p/19q co-deletion and IDH1/2 mutations. Therapy is administered, when indicated, by TCT followed by concomitant or adjuvant chemotherapy with temozolomide (TMZ) or procarbazine, lomustine (CCNU) and vincristine (PCV). With regard to the tumor origin, it proceeds from O2A precursors. IDH1/2 mutations, 1p/19q co-deletion and TERT mutations are steps of the malignant progression. Experimentally, candidates to be the cell of origins are NG2 precursor cells.

Chapter 2 – Oliogodendroglial tumours arise from oligodendroglial cells or their precursors. Typically located in cerebral hemispheres, they are diffusely infiltrating neoplasms, either well differentiated or with focal or diffuse features of malignancy. Oligodendrogliomas represent the third most common glial tumour and account for 5% of primary brain neoplasms. Besides predicting the tumour sensitivity to chemotherapy, the 1p and 19q mutations that are most frequently found in oligodendrogliomas may be useful to determine the type of tumour in morphologically ambiguous cases, as no immunohistological markers for oligodendrogliomas are known so far. In this chapter, the oligodendrogliomas and the problematic of diagnostic markers are shortly discussed.

Chapter 3 – on chromosomes 1p and 19q and the correlation of these deletions with chemoresponsiveness has had significant impact on the clinical management of these tumors and on prognosis. Some people have even gone so far as to propose that these deletions should be required to make a definitive diagnosis. The classic histologic appearance of these tumors is also somewhat distinctive – cells with rounded nuclei, absent nucleoli, scant cytoplasm and pericellular clearing (so-called fried egg appearance). From a purely morphologic perspective, however, there are a variety of other neoplasms which may have a similar appearance (look-alikes) and can potentially result in diagnostic confusion or misdiagnosis. The focus of this chapter is to examine the histopathologic differential diagnoses of oligodendroglioma and discuss features one can employ to sort through these differentials. Among the lesions to be discussed include astrocytomas and mixed gliomas, dysembryoplastic neuroepithelial tumors, neurocytomas, clear cell ependymomas, lymphomas, and pilocytic astrocytomas.

Chapter 4 – Oligodendrogliomas are diffusely infiltrating tumors that grow through white matter pathways. While these tumors are deadly in the long term and should be treated operatively whenever possible, their predisposition for eloquent tracts requires a compromise between preserving function and resecting tumor. Modern techniques of investigating functional neuroanatomy have demonstrated the variability of eloquent tracts, highlighting the misleading nature of Broca's and Wernicke's areas as fixed notions in modern neurosurgery. Given that traditional landmarks of functional neuroanatomy are too inconsistent to be used reliably in tumor patients, speech mapping is used intraoperatively to identify sites critical to language in order to preserve language function. The awake patient performs naming and other language functions with the help of a speech pathology team, while the surgeon conducts cortical and subcortical electric stimulation to map out and avoid eloquent brain areas. With this multidisciplinary care, the vast majority of patients are not harmed by surgery. Here the authors review speech mapping in oligodendroglioma operations and provide data regarding patient outcomes with these methods.

In: Oligodendrogliomas (ODs)
Editor: Chad Reeves

ISBN: 978-1-63484-278-5

Chapter 1

PATHOLOGY, MOLECULAR MECHANISMS AND CLINICAL REFERENCES OF OLIGODENDROGLIOMAS

Davide Schiffer*, Laura Annovazzi and Marta Mellai
Research Center/Policlinico di Monza Foundation, Vercelli, Italy

ABSTRACT

The chapter is based on a personal experience of 253 cases of oligodendroglial gliomas, composed of 122 grade II oligodendrogliomas (OII), 55 grade II oligodendrogliomas (OIII), 51 grade II oligoastrocytomas (OAII), 12 grade III oligoastrocytomas (OAIII) and 13 grade IV glioblastomas (GBM) with oligodendroglioma component (GBMO).

Oligodendrogliomas are more frequent in men than in women with a peak incidence of 45 years of age. In recent years, an increased incidence rate has been observed. They appear as well demarcated lesions, hypointense at T1 and hyperintense at T2 magnetic resonance imaging (MRI). Epileptic seizures and focal signs are the main clinical features.

According to the World Health Organization (WHO) classification of tumors of the central nervous system (CNS), the following histologic types can be distinguished:

* Corresponding author: davide.schiffer@unito.it.

OII. Diffuse growth and occurrence of the so-called "honeycomb" appearance and vessels with a "chicken-wire" distribution. Calcifications are frequent.

OIII. Vascular proliferation, endothelial hyperplasia and microvessel proliferation. High cell density, high number of mitoses, circumscribed necroses.

OAII. Occurrence of both an astrocytic and an oligodendroglial component. The main problem is the distinction of tumor from reactive astrocytes.

OAIII. Nuclear atypias, microvascular proliferations (MVPs), circumscribed necroses and high mitotic rate. The real existence of OA as distinct tumor entity is today denied or discussed.

GBMO. It is discussed as either glioblastoma of oligodendroglial origin, OIII or as real tumor entity.

Immunohistochemistry. It concerns multiple markers such as myelin basic protein (MBP), myelin-associated glycoprotein (MAG), PDGFRα, NG2, CNPase, MAP2, OLIG1 and OLIG2, glial fibrillary acidic protein (GFAP) and the proliferation index Ki-67/MIB-1.

Molecular genetics. Of great importance in diagnosis and prognosis, it includes 1p/19q co-deletion, somatic IDH1/2, TERT, CIC, FUBP1, TP53 and ATRX mutations, MGMT and EMP3 hypermethylation, CDKN2A/CDKN2B copy number changes.

Prognosis and therapy. The tumors are more benign than the corresponding astrocytic tumors of the same histologic grade. The prognosis depends on the grade of malignancy, histology and the genetic asset. Prognostic markers are the proliferation index Ki-67/MIB-1, 1p/19q co-deletion and IDH1/2 mutations.

Therapy is administered, when indicated, by TCT followed by concomitant or adjuvant chemotherapy with temozolomide (TMZ) or procarbazine, lomustine (CCNU) and vincristine (PCV).

With regard to the tumor origin, it proceeds from O2A precursors. IDH1/2 mutations, 1p/19q co-deletion and TERT mutations are steps of the malignant progression. Experimentally, candidates to be the cell of origins are NG2 precursor cells.

1. INTRODUCTION

The term oligodendroglioma was firstly assigned by Bailey and Bucy in agreement with the morphological similarities of tumor cells with oligodendrocytes [1]. According to the World Health Organization (WHO) classification of tumors of the central nervous system (CNS), oligodendroglial tumors are distinguished in grade II oligodendrogliomas (OII), grade III oligodendrogliomas (OIII), grade II oligoastrocytomas (OAII), grade III oligoastrocytomas (OAIII) and grade IV glioblastomas with oligodendroglial component (GBMO) [2].

1.1. The Origin of Oligodendroglioma

The current hypothesis refers to the capability of O2A precursor cells to generate oligodendroglial and astrocytic lineages [3]. On this matter, the discussion starts from the concept of glioma initiating cells (GICs). The real nature of GICs is not known; it could be due to different cell types, including oligodendrocyte precursor cells (OPCs), as it emerged from studies by the methods of mosaic analysis with double markers (MADM) [4] or by somatic cell gene transfer models [5, 6] to trace back the cell of origin.

The origin of gliomas from immature glia has long been demonstrated and the most credited theory is that they originate from neural stem cells (NSCs) of the sub-ventricular zone (SVZ) [7, 8], based, practically, on the demonstration that glioblastoma stem cells (GSCs) show the same properties of NSCs: a) the signaling pathways that regulate normal NSCs are altered in gliomas; b) GSCs are tumorigenic when transplanted into mice. Recently, another suggestion has been proposed, i.e., that OPCs are the cells of origin of gliomas [8]. The demonstration of this hypothesis is that OPCs express chondroitin sulfate or glial antigen 2 (NG2) [9], platelet-derived growth factor receptor α (PDGFRα) [10], A2B5 [11] and 2',3'-Cyclic-nucleotide 3'-phosphodiesterase (CNPase) [12]. NG2 cells are the major dividing cell population in the adult brain, being found in the SVZ, white matter, and cortex, which give origin to oligodendrocytes. Also, PDGFRα, which regulates OPC migration [13], has been found to be altered in gliomas [14]. NG2 and PDGFRα are expressed in oligodendrogliomas and OPCs can give origin to astrocytes, neurons and oligodendrocytes; by Ras activation and p53 depletion, astrocytic tumors can be elicited [15]. Recently, it has been demonstrated that in tumors induced by retroviral techniques, for instance RCAS/tv-a glioma models, OPCs, positive for NG2, resulted in being the cell of origin of gliomas [16, 17]. By a *Ctv-a* mouse model, tumor induction is restricted to OPCs expressing CNPase and this occurs in oligodendroglial cells during and after differentiation. Lindberg et al. (2009) [5] showed that PDGFβ transferred to OPCs generates gliomas resembling human OII. Committed glial progenitors can be, therefore, at their origin.

By the same RCAS/tv-a model in transgenic mice, murine oligodendrogliomas develop in association with white matter expansion of cells that show a gene expression profile typical of OPCs rather than NSCs; epidermal growth factor receptor (EGFR) expressing cells differentiate into oligodendrocytes if the mitogen-activated protein kinase (MAPK) pathway is inhibited; NG2+ and NG2- cells are sensitive to temozolomide (TMZ) and NG2+ cells are highly tumorigenic. Human oligodendrogliomas show a restricted differentiation and sphere formation, localize to white matter and express OPC markers [6]. SOX10 was also studied and found to be required for the differentiation of OPCs, favoring the genesis of gliomas [18]. Basically, immunohistochemical markers of OPCs and oligodendrogliomas would be NG2, OLIG2, PDGFRα and CNPase.

1.2. Epidemiology

Oligodendrogliomas are intracranial tumors that account for 5-25% of all gliomas and for 5-10% of all primary neoplasms. They represent >10% of all diffuse gliomas in adults and even less in children [19]. They are more frequent in men than in women and show an average age of onset between 35 and 55 years of age with a peak incidence around 45 years [20]. OII typically develop in patients under 40 and OIII in patients over 40 years of age [21].

The adjusted incidence rate of OII ranges from 0.27 to 0.35 *per* 100,000 individuals and from 0.07-0.18 *per* 100,000 individuals for OIII [22]. However, it has been observed to have recently increased, mainly due to the more accurate diagnostic criteria towards astrocytic tumors. The incidence rate for OAII is approximately 0.1 *per* 100,000 individuals, while the incidence rate of OAIII is very variable [23]. As a matter of fact, the frequency of OIII in comparison with the total number of oligodendrogliomas varies between 3.5% and 50% while the frequency of oligoastrocytomas varies between 2% and 19% [24]. This is due to the lack of stringent diagnostic criteria for the delimitation of OIII towards OII and to the revision of oligoastrocytoma as a real tumor entity.

The etiology is yet unknown. None of the hereditary tumor syndromes is associated with oligodendroglial tumors, and familial clustering is only rarely reported [24].

The tumors generally arise in the white matter of the cerebral hemispheres with a predilection in decreasing order for frontal, parietal, temporal and occipital lobes; spinal cord and cerebellar locations are rare [25].

1.3. Clinical Features

The most important signs are represented by epileptic seizures, followed by focal signs; rarely, headache as expression of increased intracranial pressure is a symptom. Tumors involving the ventricles may cause obstructive hydrocephalus and they can disseminate through the cerebrospinal fluid. Metastases outside the CNS are rare. Rarely, the clinical picture begins as stroke-like due to intracerebral hemorrhages.

1.4. Neuroradiological Features

On computed tomography (CT), oligodendrogliomas appear as mixed density (hypo- or isodense) lesions with an extremely variable aspect after enhancement. Calcifications occur frequently, mainly at the periphery of the tumor.

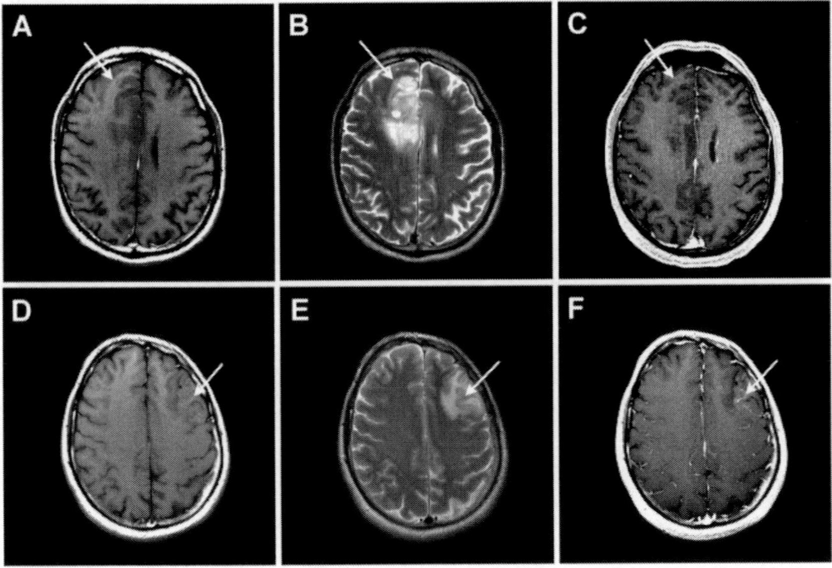

Figure 1. Magnetic resonance imaging (MRI). A – OII, hypointensity in axial T1-weighted sequence (arrow); B – OII, hyperintensity in T2-weighted sequence; C – OII, T1-weighted sequence after Gadolinium contrast enhancement; D – OIII, hypointensity in axial T1-weighted sequence (arrow); E – OIII, hyperintensity in T2-weighted sequence; F – OIII, T1-weighted sequence after Gadolinium contrast enhancement.

On magnetic resonance imaging (MRI), the tumors typically appear as round or oval marginated masses, sometimes with calcifications, more frequently hypointense in T1 and hyperintense in T2, except calcified areas. In particular, tumors with intact 1p/19q show a more homogeneous signal on T1 and T2 images and have sharper borders compared to tumors with the 1p/19q co-deletion.

Subtle ill-defined enhancement following contrast administration can occur. Contrast enhancement with Gadolinium is not rare (Figure 1A–F); it has been regarded to be proportional to tumor vasculature [26] and to occur in 50-60% of cases [27] or less [28]. According to some authors, the degree of contrast enhancement is not a reliable indicator of tumor grade [27], but, according to others, a greater number of OIII shows enhancement in comparison with OII [28]. Maybe the brain blood barrier (BBB) disruption also contributes to it.

Diffusion-weighted MRI (DWI), expressed by the apparent diffusion coefficient (ADC) parameter, has been found to be useful in differentiating high and low grade tumors, since it is associated with cellularity [28, 29]. Also, calcifications seem to be more frequent in OIII than in OII, but not in a significant way. It has not be ascertained whether the relative cerebral blood volume (rCBV) value increases [30, 31] or not [32, 33]; it seems to increase in low grade tumors with 1p/19q loss [30].

Peritumor edema is minimal and necroses can be present. Rarely, the tumor is intra-ventricular or shows diffusion into *cisternae* and subarachnoid spaces [34]. By conventional 2-[18F]-fluoro-2-deoxy-D-glucose (^{18}F-FDG)-positron emission tomography (PET), ^{18}F-FDG uptake may be similar to the uptake of the white matter in OII and to that of the gray matter in OIII [28].

2. PATHOLOGY

2.1. Macroscopic Appearance

Macroscopically, the tumors show as infiltrating the cortex from the white matter. They may acquire a gray-reddish color and show a "garland" appearance due to the growth in the subarachnoid space with re-invasion of the brain. Frequently, the tumor may invade the ventricles. Areas of mucoid degeneration, cystic changes and intra-tumor hemorrhages are not unusual.

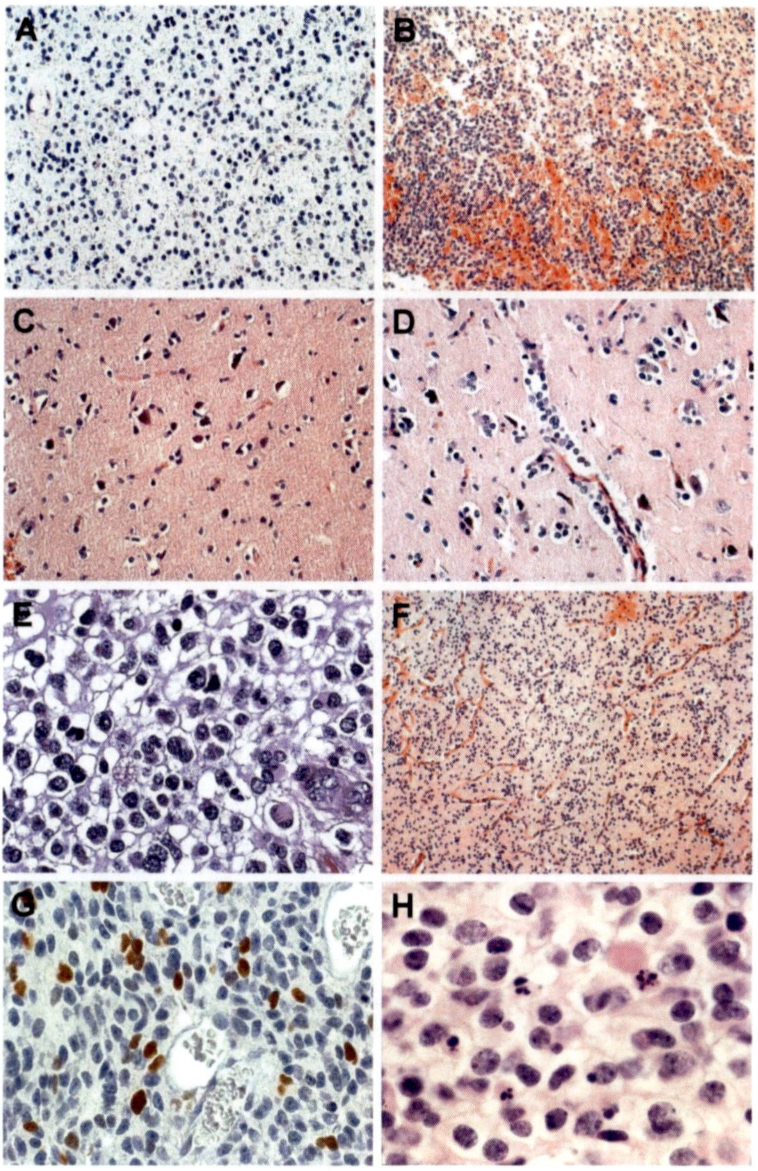

Figure 2. Histopathologic fetaures of OII. A – Low cell density, H&E, x200; B – Nodular growth pattern, H&E, x100; C – Mild infiltration, H&E, x200; D – Pericapillary tumor cells, H&E, x200; E – Typical honeycomb pattern, H&E, x400; F – Chicken-wire branching capillaries, H&E, x100; G – Ki-67/MIB-1 proliferation index, DAB, x400; H – Apoptotic nuclei, H&E, x630.

2.2. Microscopic Appearance

OII

The tumor shows a low or moderate cell density (Figure 2A) with a rare nodular growth (Figure 2B) and often a diffuse infiltration pattern (Figure 2C) with an increased number of pericapillary cells in the white matter (Figure 2D). The cells have round and hyperchromatic nuclei with a typical chromatin distribution and, frequently, a perinuclear "halo" (Figure 2E) realizing the so-called "honeycomb" or "fried eggs" appearance. The vessels show a delicate branching with a typical "chicken-wire" distribution (Figure 2F). Mitoses are rare and the labeling index (LI) for the proliferation marker Ki-67/MIB-1 is usually <10%, although higher values are not rare (Figure 2G) [25]. Apoptotic nuclei occur in greater amount compared to astrocytic tumors (Figure 2H) [35].

The so-called calcifications, i.e., pseudocalcium-calcium (pCa-Ca) precipitations, are frequent (Figure 3A). Endothelial hyperplasia and microvascular proliferations (MVPs) can occur (Figure 3B, C). Reactive astrocytes are frequent and they remain long visible in the advancing tumor parenchyma (Figure 3D, E). Infiltration in the cortex is frequent, with tumors cells crowding around neurons, especially in the Vth layer, to form the so-called "perineuronal satellitosis" in which the number of satellite cells increases from one to many (Figure 3F). Another typical feature is the crowding of tumor cells in the sub-pial region.

Sometimes, nuclei may assume a typical distribution similar to rosettes or rhythmic palisadings as in "polar spongioblastoma" (Figure 3G) [36]. Perivascular lymphocytic infiltrates are not rare (Figure 3H).

OIII

Compared to OII, the tumor shows a higher cell density (Figure 4A) and a more frequent nodular growth, increased number of mitoses (Figure 4B) or Ki-67/MIB-1 LI (Figure 4C), nuclear atypias (Figure 4B), endothelial hyperplasia and MVPs or glomeruli (Figure 4D), proliferative vascular walls (Figure 4E) and necroses with or without pseudopalisading (Figure 4F). Microcalcifications may also be present. The focal or diffuse occurrence of one or more of these histologic features may indicate anaplasia, but, practically, things are not so simple, because sometimes they can also be individually found in OII. By multivariate analysis, they do not significantly indicate grade III [37]. A crucial finding is the number of mitoses or of Ki-67/MIB-1 positive nuclei. For instance, >6 mitoses *per* 10 high power field

(HPF) would indicate OIII [38]. The cut-off value of the Ki-67/MIB-1 LI between OII and OIII is very high since a grade II tumor tolerates up to 15% positive nuclei [25]. This is very important, since the grading *criteria* are different between oligodendrogliomas and astrocytomas; the same glioma would be classified as grade II or III with the same Ki-67/MIB-1 LI according to the histologic diagnosis [39].

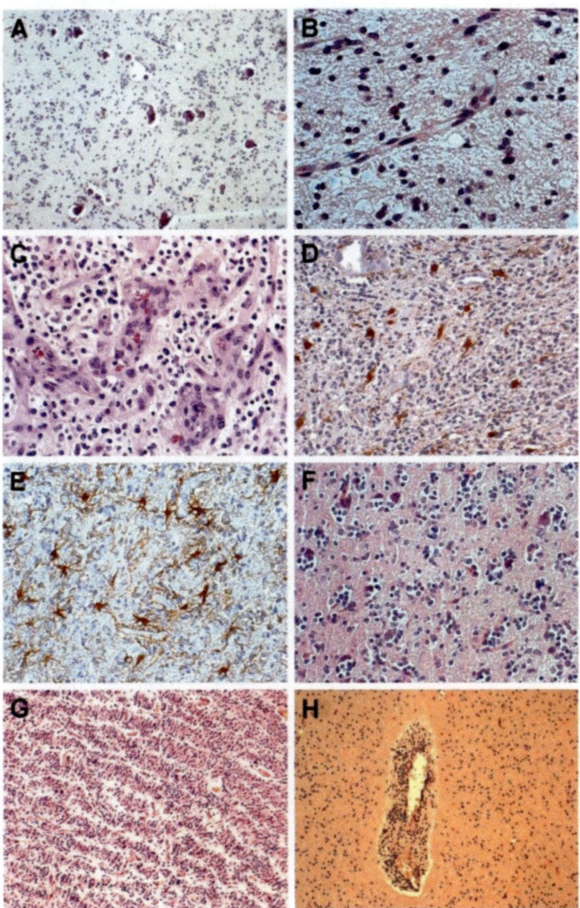

Figure 3. Histopathologic features of OII. A – Calcifications, H&E, x100; B – Endothelial hyperplasia, H&E, x400; C – Microvascular proliferations, H&E, x200; D – GFAP-positive reactive astrocytes inside the tumor, DAB, x200; E – GFAP-positive reactive astrocytes outside the tumor, DAB, x200; F – Cortical perineuronal satellitosis, H&E, x200; G – Rhythmic palisadings, H&E, x100; H – Perivascular lymphocytic infiltrates, H&E, x100.

The same thing is true for MVPs and necroses that indicate grade IV in astrocytic tumors and still grade III in oligodendroglioma, taking into account that they can occur even in tumors with an overall survival (OS) typical of OII [25]. It has been confirmed that they do not indicate necessarily a poor prognosis in OIII [40]. The discussion of this matter would involve the existence of either an OIV or a GBMO [41].

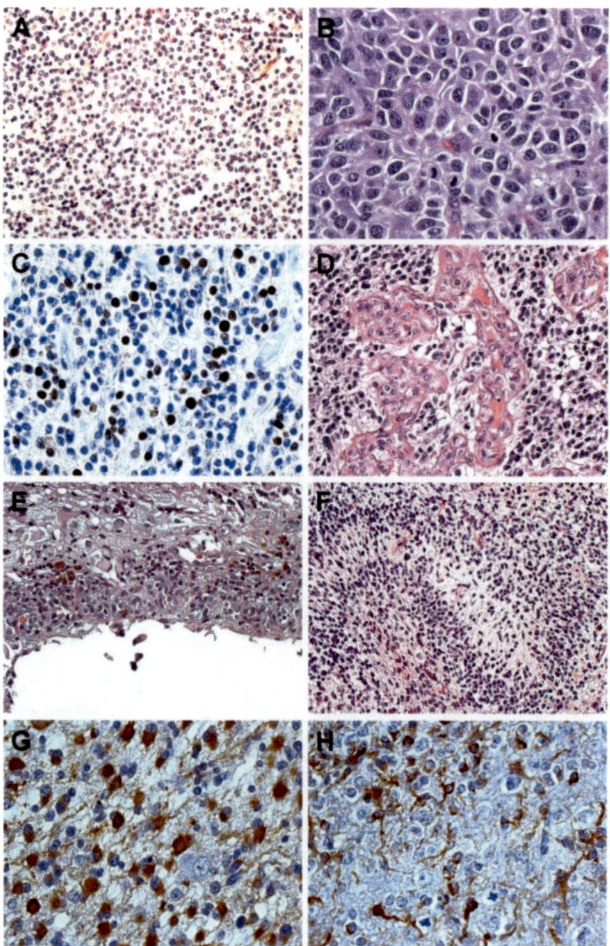

Figure 4. Histopathologic features of OIII. A – High cell density, H&E, x100; B – Nuclear atypias and mitoses, H&E, x400; C – Ki-67/MIB-1 proliferation index, DAB, x400; D – Glomeruli, H&E, x400; E – Proliferative vascular wall, DAB, x200; F – Circumscribed necrosis, H&E, x200; G – GFAP-positive round minigemistocytes, DAB, x400; H – GFAP-positive gliofibrillary oligodendrocytes (GFOC), DAB, x400.

A particular finding, which can also occur in OII and not be regarded as a marker of malignancy, eventhough some may consider it of ominous meaning, is represented by the so-called minigemistocytes (Figure 4G), with a round glial fibrillary acidic protein (GFAP)+ cytoplasm without processes and a peripheral nucleus, and by the so-called gliofibrillary oligodendrocyes (GFOCs) (Figure 4H). The former have been interpreted as small gemistocytes without gliofibrils [42] or transitional cells between oligodendrocytes and astrocytes [43] or corresponding to bipotential precursors [44] or as expression of transition forms [45], reminiscent of the myelin forming glia [46].

OAII

The tumor contains both an astrocytic and an oligodendroglial component (Figure 5A, B), which may be either diffusely intermingled or separated into distinct areas. They are quantitatively variable so that the differential diagnosis towards astrocytomas and oligodendrogliomas remains difficult. The problem does not exist when the two components are clearly separated, but this rarely happens. Usually, the tumor appears as containing scattered astrocytes in an oligodendroglial context. There is no doubt that GFAP+ astrocytes exist in oligodendroglial tumors, either as minigemistocytes or GFOCs or reactive astrocytes with thick and long processes. The most important problem is to precisely differentiate tumor astrocytes from reactive astrocytes. Usually, reactive astrocytes are distributed at a regular distance from one another, respecting their proxemics law. They can be found in the peritumor normal tissue or entrapped in the tumor where they can be distinguished from tumor astrocytes for their size and broader processes; they can also be smaller and numerous when they are recently formed. The aspect of their nuclei is different from the aspect of tumor oligodendrocytes. The detection of small reactive or tumor astrocytes is easier in the tumor than in its invasion area where large reactive astrocytes are clearly visible.

Another problem is represented by the percentage of oligodendrocytes or of astrocytes necessary for the diagnosis [47]. Ten percent of oligodendrocytes [48] or astrocytes [49] have been proposed. Not last, the possibility must be contemplated that a tumor is an astrocytoma infiltrating the white matter in which oligodendrocytes mimics an oligodendroglial component. These are the reasons for the wide variability in the diagnosis of oligoastrocytomas, on which more will be said later.

OAIII

The tumor is mainly characterized by an increased mitotic activity; it should be decided whether it occurs in the oligodendroglial or in the astrocytic component. Usually, when the last one occurs, a more aggressive treatment is suggested [40, 50], since OAIII with necroses has a shorter survival time. The problem is the differential diagnosis towards GBMs when necrosis affects the astrocytic component, whereas the occurrence of MVPs does not favor the diagnosis of AOIII when they occur in the oligodendroglial component. OAII and OAIII have been put in doubt as tumor variants after the discovery of somatic mutations in the thalassemia/mental retardation syndrome X-linked (ATRX) gene (see later).

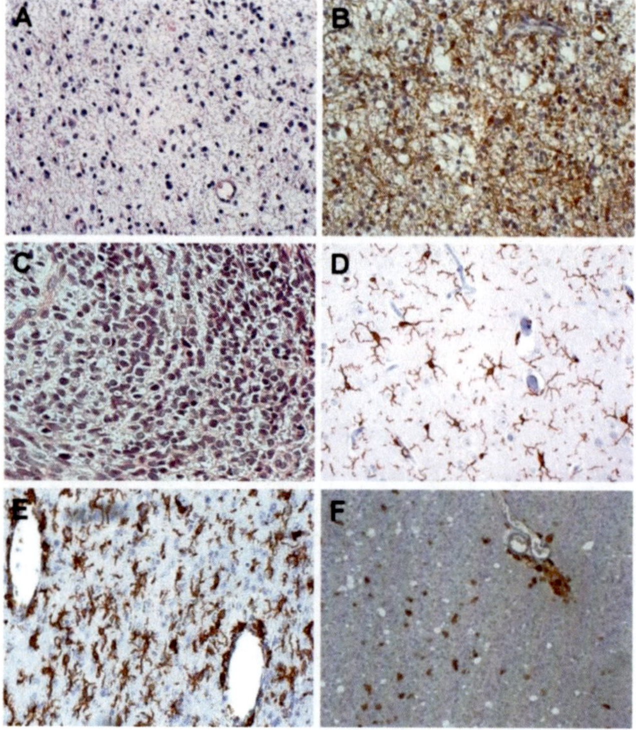

Figure 5. OAII, GBMO, TAMs. A – OAII, H&E, x200; B – OAII, GFAP-positive tumor cells, DAB, x200; C – GBMO, H&E, x400; D – OII, Iba1-positive ramified microglia cells in mildly infiltrated cortex, DAB, x200; E – OII, Iba1-positive reactive microglia with coarse processes and perivascular macrophages, DAB, x200; F – OII, perivascular and scattered CD163-positive reactive microglia, DAB, x100.

GBMO

Primary GBMO is recognized as a subgroup of GBMs classified as a grade IV tumor entity; it resembles OAIII with necroses. The tumor shows histologic features of GBM in which circumscribed areas with typical oligodendroglial characteristics, such as, for instance, the "honeycomb" appearance, are found. Circumscribed necroses, calcifications and cystic components may be present as well (Figure 5C) [51].

GBMO accounts for approximately 5-20% of all GBMs and it associates with a younger age at diagnosis [52]. When present, honeycomb-like features and pseudopalisading necrosis have a prognostic significance [51].

Currently, GBMO is not regarded as a tumor variant, but, rather, as a pattern of differentiation [2]. The differential diagnosis is towards OIII and OAIII.

2.3. Microglia/Macrophages

Human gliomas show prominent infiltration of microglia/macrophages, which correlates with the grade of malignancy. In GBMs, the number of microglia/macrophages or tumor-associated macrophages (TAMs) or glioblastoma-associated macrophages (GAMs) is higher than in grade II or III gliomas and it is closely correlated with the vascular density in the tumor [53, 54]. Infiltrating GAMs may account for up to 30% of the tumor mass. Cyclooxygenase (Cox) 1 and 2 and heme oxygenase 1 (Ho-1) expression have been shown to mark GAMs in gliomas and to increase in relapsing oligodendrogliomas, especially around necroses and in the peritumor tissue [55, 56]. In other experiences, the ionized calcium-binding adaptor molecule 1 (Iba1)-positive GAMs of the tumor core of OIII were significantly more activated than Iba1-positive microglia of non-neoplastic brain tissue. Iba1 expression showed a positive correlation with Ki-67/MIB-1 expression in all gliomas. Most TAMs showed a rarer expression of CD68, CD163 or CD204, although CD204-positive TAMs were mainly observed in necroses, as well as in the proliferative vascular walls [57].

Based on the classical distinction of M1 and M2 cells, corresponding respectively to pro-inflammatory or pro-tumor cells, several studies demonstrated that CD163 is a marker of M2 macrophages [58–61], especially when combined with CD68 and c-MAF, even though combinations of M1 and M2 co-exist in the immune cell responses [62].

By using CD68, Iba1, CD16 and CD163 antibodies, which differently depict normal resident or reactive ramified microglia, amoeboid microglia and macrophages originating from the blood borne monocyte phagocytic cells, it was observed that Iba1+ microglia cells increase from the normal cortex to tumor infiltration, showing progressively thick and coarse processes (Figure 5 D, E); in the tumor core, Iba1 immunopositivity depicts the round and granular aspect of macrophages. CD68 immunostaining depicts the cells with small granules along the processes and with coarse grains in ameboid microglia or macrophages. In fact, in the tumor core, macrophages prevail on ramified microglia cells. CD16 and Iba1 share a similar immunostaining pattern, whereas CD163 preferentially marks macrophages, but, irregularly, also ramified microglia (Figure 5F). c-MAF would perhaps distinguish a CD68 sub-population with M2 function [62]. Passage forms exist between ramified microglia and true macrophages. It has been demonstrated that the GAM phenotype only shows partial overlap with M1, M2a, M2b, and M2c phenotypes. For instance, GAMs do not fit into a classical M1 or M2 phenotype, but represent a unique phenotype: some GAMs are polarized towards a M1-like phenotype, whereas other GAMs possess a more M2-like phenotype, and still another population of GAMs is not polarized towards M1 or M2-like states. Therefore, single-cell sequencing of GAMs would help to better understand their activation status [63].

TAMs/GAMs are still under discussion, whether they are “friend” or “foe” [64], i.e., which action prevails between the pro-tumor or the inflammatory anti-tumor function.

2.4. Differential Diagnosis and Prognosis

To date, no truly specific immunohistochemical marker exists for oligodendroglial tumors. The many proposed until now are undoubtedly positive in oligodendroglial tumors but they can also do so in other neoplastic conditions: myelin basic protein (MBP), myelin-associated glycoprotein (MAG), PDGFRα, NG2, CNPase, MAP2, OLIG1 and OLIG2 [24]. We have already discussed GFAP+ cells in oligodendrogliomas.

Clinical parameters have been identified for the prediction of patient outcome. In particular, age at surgery, extent of surgical resection, frontal location, post-operative Karnofsky score and lack of contrast enhancement are associated with prognosis by both uni- and multivariate analysis [25].

Histopathologic parameters associated with a worse prognosis include increased cellularity, high mitotic activity, nuclear atypia and cellular polymorphism, MVPs and necroses [25]. However, in contrast to astrocytic tumors, the occurrence of MVPs and necroses alone does not imply the clinical outcome of OIII.

The problem of the distinction of astrocytomas from oligodendrogliomas seems to have been solved by the new acquisitions; however, some doubts persist about oligoastrocytomas. The tissue events to be considered are: a) the prevailing aspect of diffuse and infiltrative growth of oligodendrogliomas and of the oligodendroglial component of oligoastrocytomas; b) the occurrence of reactive astrocytes, the distribution and size of which depends on their age, and of small tumor astrocytes with uncertainty about their GFAP immunostaining; c) the occurrence of the so-called minigemistocytes and large gemistocytes; d) the occurrence of normal oligodendrocytes, either as perineural satellites in the cortex or as the major cell component of the white matter; e) the possibility to interpret these oligodendrocytes in an infiltrating astrocytoma as the oligodendroglial component of oligoastrocytomas; f) mainly, the knowledge that missense mutations of ATRX have no effect on the protein expression; g) not all astrocytic tumors show lack of ATRX protein expression/ATRX mutations and, finally, h) ATRX is expressed in neurons and in microglia, infiltrating and endothelial cells, but not in normal astro- and oligodendroglia.

Differential diagnosis assumes a special importance when it must be done on very small surgical samples, for instance on stereotactic biopsies, and when a therapeutic strategy has to be chosen. It mainly concerns infiltrating oligodendroglioma *versus* normal white matter; oligodendroglioma *versus* diffuse astrocytoma; OII *versus* OIII, and OIII *versus* GBMO. The distinction of oligodendroglioma infiltrating cells from normal white matter oligodendrocytes can be very difficult when the infiltration is very mild. The nuclear morphology may be of help and quantitative cytophotometric methods on Feulgen-stained sections have been proposed [65], but they are too complicated for surgical pathology. The increase of perineuronal satellites in the near cortex or of pericapillary satellites in the white matter is more helpful. At worst, cell counts can be used.

The distinction between OII and AII can be difficult and this is proved by the complementarity of the two diagnoses in the different series, i.e., when the frequency of oligodendrogliomas increases, that of astrocytomas decreases [48, 66]. Practically, it is based on cytological characteristics [48, 67, 68]. The danger in confusing the two tumors resides in the different biological significance of the same tissue events. The same value of the Ki-67/MIB-1 LI has different meanings in the two tumors, indicating anaplasia in astrocytomas when >10%, but not in oligodendrogliomas [47]. The distinction of normal oligodendrocytes from a mild tumor infiltration can be achieved exploiting the positivity of the former for Cyclin D1, dissociated from Cyclin A and B1, and the negativity of the latter [69]. However, this cannot be used in OIII, because Cyclin D1 expression increases in cycling cells [70]. In contrast, OLIG1 is not considered as specific marker for oligodendroglia, being positive also in astrocytomas [71, 72]. It has been found positive in GFOCs, but negative in minigemistocytes [73]. The same thing is true for OLIG2 [74] and MAP2 [75].

The distinction of OII *versus* OIII is often difficult. In multivariate analysis, circumscribed necroses, endothelial hyperplasia, MVPs and high vessel density did not result in prognostic factors, although they were more frequent in OIII. The only *criterion* is the Ki-67/MIB-1 LI that, however, must be very high to indicate OIII [37, 47], since OII tolerates values much higher compared to AII. It is a useful marker to distinguish between OII and OIII, but with a cut-off value approximately >20% of positive nuclei.

In most cases, the diagnosis of OIII is straightforward. In a fraction of cases, however, the diagnosis *versus* OAIII is problematic and associated with a considerable degree of interobserver variability. The distinction of highly cellular and poorly differentiated OIII from malignant astrocytic neoplasms may be facilitated by molecular genetics analysis. Interestingly, considering both histologic and molecular features on a large series of 203 OIII, three groups were histologically identified among 1p/19q co-deleted cases associated with molecular differences: 1) OIII with >5 mitoses/10 HPF without MVPs and necroses; 2) OIII with MVP and no necroses; 3) OIII with both MVPs and necroses [76].

A great problem is represented by the differential diagnosis between OAII and OAIII. Their frequency greatly varies in the different collections, since there are no stringent *criteria* for the diagnosis. The recent discovery of ATRX mutations, responsible for the lack of ATRX protein expression, provided new insights to improve the conventional histologic classification. Following recent revisions, tumors should be regarded either as oligodendrogliomas or astrocytomas, being the astrocytic component composed of reactive astrocytes [77, 78], although not by everybody [79]. In our experience, we agree that most oligoastrocytomas should be classified either as oligodendrogliomas or astrocytomas, but some oligoastrocytomas seem to exist, since the astrocytic component is not always reactive (personal unpublished data).

Finally, oligodendrogliomas need to be distinguished from macrophage-rich reactive lesions (demyelinating diseases or cerebral strokes), as well as from other tumor types that may present with clear cells, for instance clear cell ependymoma, neurocytoma, dysembryoplastic neuroepithelial tumor (DNET), clear cell meningioma, and metastatic clear cell carcinoma. In this regard, immunohistochemical analysis usually is useful to separate these tumor entities.

As for GBMO, it is not difficult to recognize the oligodendroglial component. It is difficult to interpret it, provided that the oligodendroglial component is not formed by normal oligodendrocytes of the white matter.

3. Molecular Genetics with Reference to Differential Diagnosis and Prognosis

Beside morphology [2], three genetic events seem to characterize low grade gliomas: recurrent somatic point mutations of the isocitrate dehydrogenase (IDH) 1 and 2 genes [80–82], 1p/19q co-deletion, mainly marking oligodendrogliomas and excluding astrocytomas [83, 84], TERT promoter mutations or ATRX mutations [85]. More recently, it has been demonstrated that the 1p/19q co-deletion associates with IDH1/2 mutations to mark oligodendrogliomas [81], whereas TP53 and ATRX are the only genetic events to mark astrocytomas [86].

3.1. 1p/19q Chromosomal Status

The genetic hallmark of oligodendroglial tumors is a combined chromosomal deletion of the short arm of the chromosome 1 (1p) and the long arm of the chromosome 19 (19q). The 1p/19q co-deletion is usually present in up to 80% of OII and in 50-70% of OIII [83, 87].

The 1p/19q chromosomal status is useful in clinical practice as an important diagnostic biomarker. The 1p/19q co-deletion is typical of oligodendrogliomas with a classical histologic phenotype (perinuclear "halo" and "chicken-wire" vascular pattern), whereas tumors without it more frequently show astrocytic features [88, 89]. Oligodendroglial tumors with 1p/19q co-deletion typically occur at an extratemporal location, whereas tumors with intact 1p/19q prevail in the temporal lobe [87]. It has been observed that the apoptotic index (AI) is higher in oligodendrogliomas harboring 1p/19q co-deletion compared to tumors with intact 1p/19q [90]. This can be explained not only by the different clinical behavior, but also by the higher AI in oligodendrogliomas compared to astrocytomas, and by the frequent uncertainty in the differential diagnosis between the two glioma types [37, 91]. The 1p/19q co-deletion could be more reliable in the diagnosis than morphology [92] and this could also explain its lower frequency in OIII, being the differentiation of the latter from GBMs not so certain. The occurrence of 1p/19q co-deletion supports the diagnosis of oligodendroglioma particularly when the histologic findings are atypical. However, its absence does not exclude this diagnosis, leaving the question of oligodendrogliomas with intact 1p/19q unsolved.

When present, the 1p/19q co-deletion is generally distributed through the tumor also in areas with a more astrocytic morphology [93]. Moreover, it is retained at the time of progression, regardless of morphologic changes [94].

In oligoastrocytomas, the rate of the 1p/19q co-deletion is in the range of 50% [87]. Virtually, it is mutually exclusive with the loss of heterozygosity (LOH) on chromosome 17p13 and with TP53 somatic mutations, both typical of astrocytic tumors. In oligoastrocytomas, the 1p/19q co-deletion refers to the oligodendroglial component, whereas TP53 mutations to the astrocytic one. This finding indicates a clonal origin of oligoastrocytomas and supports the hypothesis of two genetic assets deriving from different tumor locations. Interestingly, TP53 mutations prevail in temporal oligoastrocytomas rather than in extratemporal tumors [87].

In GBMO, the 1p/19q co-deletion has been reported with a similar or even higher frequency compared to GBMs [51, 95]. When detected in GBMs, it may suggest a diagnosis of GBMO [96].

The 1p/19q co-deletion has also been described in both the glial and sarcomatous components of gliosarcoma [97].

3.2. Mechanism of the Combined Loss of Chromosomes 1p and 19q

The mechanism of the combined loss of the two chromosomal arms is an unbalanced t(1;19)(q10;p10) translocation of 19p to 1q [98, 99]. Probably, a centromeric or pericentromeric translocation of chromosomes 1 and 19 results in two derivative chromosomes, der(1;19)(p10;q10) and der(1;19)(q10;p10), followed by the loss of the derivative chromosome containing the short arm of chromosome 1 and the long arm of chromosome 19 (Figure 6).

A possible explanation for the translocation is the strong sequence homology of the centromeric region of chromosomes 1 and 19, which may promote instability and translocation events [99]. The translocation has been described in approximately 90% of cases with demonstrated 1p/19q loss [99]. The 1p/19q co-deletion has been reported in short-term culture of oligodendroglioma also without evidence of t(1;19)(q10;p10) translocation [100].

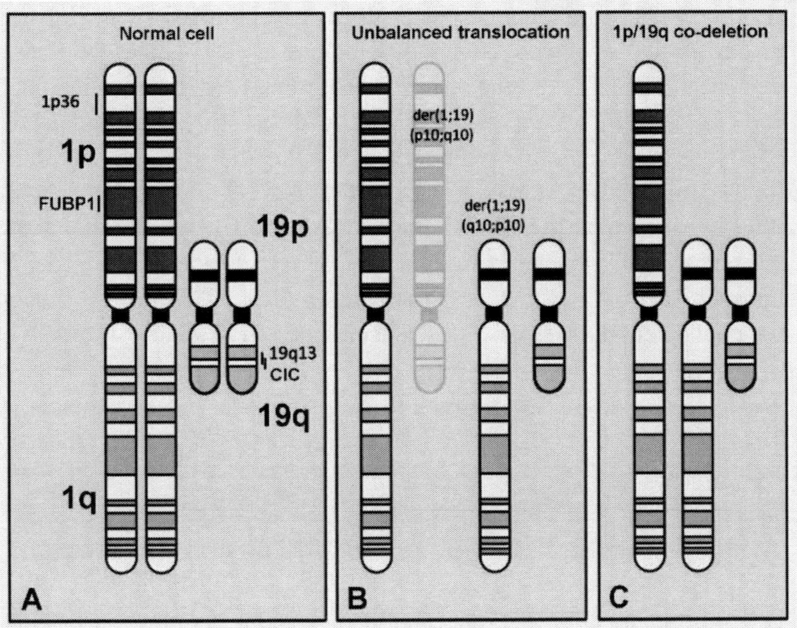

Figure 6. Model for t(1;19)(q10;p10) translocation mechanism in oligodendroglial tumors according to Griffin et al. [98] (modified from Ref. 232). A – Normal cells contain two copies of the chromosomes 1 and 19, each with a short (p) arm and a long (q) arm. The location of FUBP1 (1p31.1) and CIC (19q13.2) genes are indicated, as well as the most commonly used probes on 1p36 and 19q13 by fluorescent *in situ* hybridization (FISH). B – Unbalanced translocation leads to the formation of the derivative chromosome der(1;19)(p10;q10) (left, shaped) and its subsequent loss and to the derivative chromosome der(1,19)(q10;p10). C – The loss of chromosomal arms 1p and 19q results in one copy of 1p and 19q and in two copies of 1q and 19p.

The extent of the 1p/19q co-deletion has great diagnostic and prognostic implications. The entire chromosomal arm 1p is typically deleted only in oligodendroglial tumors and has a strong favorable prognostic significance. However, small telomeric or interstitial 1p deletions are frequent as well, in particular at the cytogenetic band 1p36, but they have an opposite prognostic significance and associate neither with deletion on the chromosomal arm 19q [101] nor with response to CHT [102]. With regard to the 19q chromosomal arm, the deletion is typically analyzed at the cytogenetic band 19q13. Isolated 1p and 19q deletions are frequently observed also in astrocytic gliomas, in relation with the malignant transformation [103]. Partial 1p deletions are frequent in GBMs, while partial 19q deletions prevail in AIII [104].

To date, the scientific community agrees to recognize the classical oligodendroglioma based on the occurrence of a total 1p/19q co-deletion [105, 106].

Most oligodendrogliomas with 1p/19q co-deletion harbor somatic IDH1/2, TERT, CIC and FUBP1 mutations, as well as MGMT or CDKN2A ($p14^{ARF}$) promoter hypermethylations. In contrast, LOH on 17p13 and TP53 mutations are rare and mutually exclusive with the 1p/19q co-deletion, as well LOH on chromosome 10q or EGFR gene amplification [105, 107–109]. Virtually all 1p/19q co-deleted tumors have a Proneural gene expression profile [110], supporting the hypothesis that oligodendrogliomas arise from bipotential progenitor cells able to give origin to both neurons and oligodendrocytes [110].

3.3. Methods for the Detection of 1p/19q Chromosomal Status

Different methods for the detection of the 1p/19q chromosomal status are currently employed in the routine diagnostics. Conventional diagnostic techniques such as LOH analysis with microsatellite markers or fluorescent *in situ* hybridization (FISH) both allow single-locus analyses, typically limited to the 1p36 locus, but they do not discriminate between total *versus* partial 1p deletions [102, 105, 111]. In contrast, multi-locus techniques such as comparative genomic hybridization (CGH) or multiplex ligation-dependent amplification (MLPA) provide complementary information to assess the 1p/19q chromosomal status [112]. These techniques detect gene copy number changes and may identify putative gain of functions on chromosomes 1p and 19q [113–115]. Recently, MLPA has been validated as a high-resolution gene dosage assay for the screening of large deletions and duplication/amplification events in human cancers. In particular, three independent studies proved the usefulness of MLPA for the assessment of the 1p/19q status in gliomas by comparing MLPA data with CGH or FISH data obtained on the same tumor series, mainly composed of oligodendroglial tumors [115–117].

3.4. Candidate Tumor Suppressor Genes (TSGs) on 1p and 19q

An interesting question concerns the existence of putative TSGs on chromosomes 1p and 19q that could be important in the origin of oligodendrogliomas.

Candidate TSGs on chromosome 1p include SHREW1 (1p36.32) [118], TP73 (1p36.32) [118], DFFB (1p36.32) [118, 119], CAMTA1 (1p36.31-1p36.23) [102], CITED4 (1p34.2) [120], RAD54 (1p34.1) [121], CDKN2C (1p32.3) [122, 123], DIRAS3 (1p31.3) [124], FUBP1 (1p31.1) [107] and NOTCH2 (1p12-p11) [125]. Notably, NOTCH2 is the most centromeric gene and mapping studies would indicate that the most frequent translocation breakpoint maps are within this gene [125].

Contrary to the chromosomal region 1p, the loss of which is associated with the unique clinical phenotype of 1p/19q co-deleted oligodendroglial tumors, the search for TSGs on the candidate region 19q was mainly focused on astrocytic tumors with partial deletion. With regard to the chromosome 19q, the putative TSGs include ZNF342/296 (19q13.32) [126], p190R_{ho}GAP (19q13.3) [127], EMP3 (19q13.33) [120, 128], PEG3 (19q.13.43) [123] and CIC (19q13.2) [107].

To date, definitive evidence for any of these candidate genes has yet to be demonstrated.

3.5. IDH1/2 Mutations

IDHs catalyze the oxidative decarboxylation of isocitrate to α-ketoglutarate with production of NADH/NADPH and they are involved in the Krebs cycle.

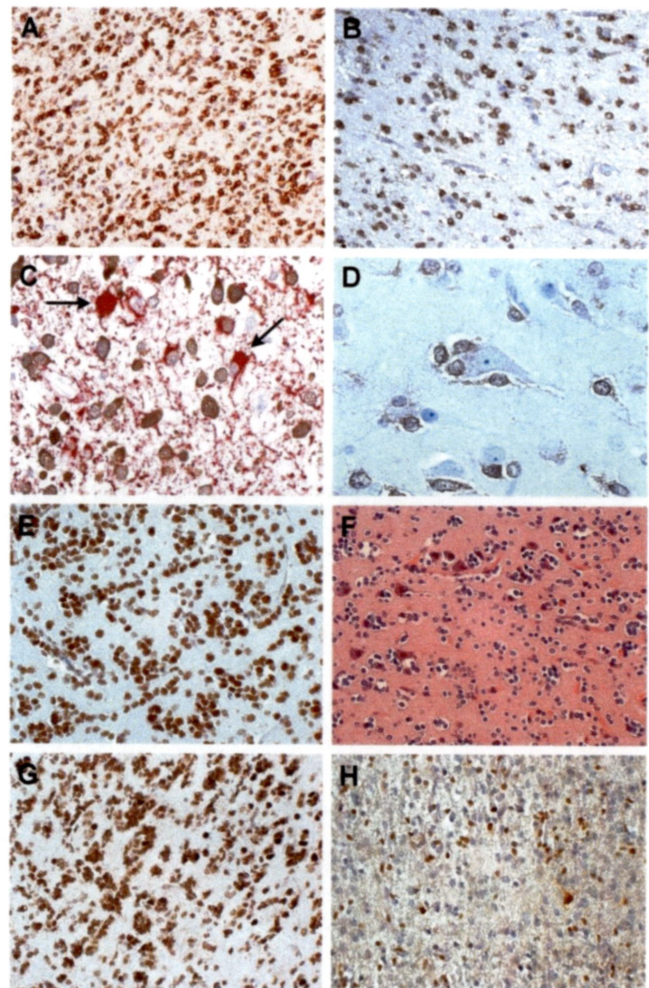

Figure 7. Anti-IDH1^{R132H} mouse monoclonal antibody (clone H09, Dianova GmbH, Hamburg, Germany) immunohistochemistry (IHC): A – OIII, positive perinuclear rim in tumor cells, DAB, x200; B – OIII, negative normal and positive tumor oligodendrocytes in the infiltrated white matter, DAB, 200x; C – OIII, IDH1^{R132H}-positive tumor cells and GFAP-positive reactive astrocytes (arrows), double IHC with DAB and *Fast Red*, respectively, x400; D – OII, positive cortical perineuronal satellites, DAB, x400. Anti-ATRX rabbit polyclonal antibody (HPA001906, Sigma Aldrich Co., St. Louis, MO, USA) IHC: E – OII, positive nuclei in the tumor core, DAB, x200; F – OII, cortical infiltration and satellitosis, H&E, x200; G – OII, intensely positive nuclei of tumor cells in the cortical infiltration, DAB, x200; H – OAII, positive and negative nuclei of tumor cells, DAB, x200.

Recurrent somatic point mutations affect the arginine (Arg) residue at codon 132 in the IDH1 gene on chromosome 2q33.3. Less frequently, they occur at the homolog Arg residue at codon 172 in the IDH2 gene on chromosome 15q26.1. The IDH1/2 mutation rate is 70-80% in OII and OIII [81, 82, 129, 130] and less in OAII and OAIII, with a higher frequency in 1p/19q co-deleted tumors [105]. IDH1 mutations prevail in astrocytic tumors whereas IDH2 mutations typically prevail in oligodendroglial tumors [82, 132].

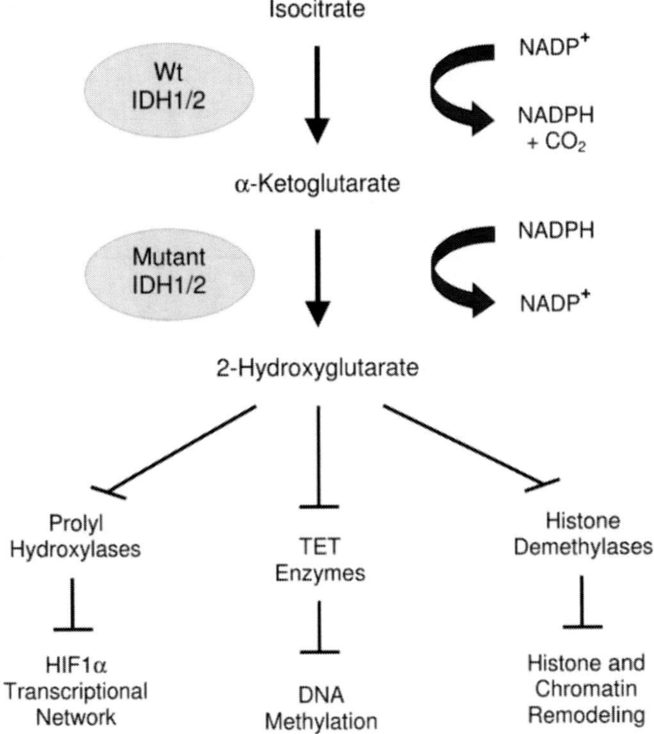

Figure 8. Functions of wild type and mutant isocitrate dehydrogenases (IDH) 1 and 2 (modified from Ref .181). The wild type IDH1/2 isoforms catalyze the oxidative decarboxylation of isocitrate to α-ketoglutarate (α-KG) in the Krebs cycle and generates nicotinamide adenine dinucleotide phosphate (NADPH). In contrast, cancer-associated IDH1/2 mutations exhibit an altered substrate specificity that results in the production of the oncometabolite D-2-hydroxyglutarate (D-2-HG). The accumulation of 2-HG inhibits prolyl-hydroxylases, TET enzymes and histone demethylases, leading to inactivation of the hypoxia-inducible factor 1 α (HIF-1α) pathway and to aberrant epigenetic modifications in tumor cells.

In low-grade gliomas, they are prognostically favorable factors [130, 133, 134]. The c.395G > A (p.R132H) mutation can be easily detected by a mutant-specific anti-$IDH1^{R132H}$ antibody by immunohistochemical techniques [130, 131]. Most tumor cells show $IDH1^{R132H}$ immunopositivity in their cytoplasms (Figure 7A, B), whereas reactive astrocytes and normal glia cells are negative (Figure 7C). This is particularly evident in the picture of cortical perineuronal satellitosis ((Figure 7D) where, when the cortical invasion begins, positive (tumor) and negative (normal) satellites can be found.

IDH1/2 mutations afford a gain of function to tumor cells. In fact, they are responsible for metabolic alterations, including an increased production of 2-hydroxyglutarate (2-HG) that can impair histone demethylation and induce a glioma-CpG island methylator phenotype (G-CIMP) [135, 136] (Figure 8).

$IDH1^{R132H}$ and ATRX immunohistochemistry (IHC), followed by subsequent copy number analysis and IDH1/2 sequencing has been proposed as a basis for an “integrated” diagnostic approach for adult oligodendrogliomas [106].

3.6. Telomerase Reverse Transcriptase (TERT) Promoter Mutations

The human telomerase is a structurally complex ribonucleoprotein responsible for the maintenance of telomeric DNA at the ends of chromosomes. It has an important role in cell immortalization and in oncogenesis. In particular, TERT elongates telomeres by adding hexameric 5’-TTAGGG-3’ tandem repeats at chromosomal ends. In somatic cells, telomeres shorten at each cycle of cell division [137] and, beyond a critical point, cells undergo senescence and apoptosis [138]. In malignant tumors, including gliomas, telomerase is reactivated and cells escape telomere shortening [139]. Two main and mutually exclusive C228T and C250T point mutations are located in the core promoter region of the TERT gene, both associated with increased TERT expression and telomerase activity [140–142]. They were first reported in melanomas and in a variety of human neoplasms, including gliomas [143].

In the latter, TERT promoter mutations associated with oligodendroglioma diagnosis in an older age, are more frequent in high (75.8%) than in low grade tumors (45.9%) and in oligodendrogliomas (64.2%) than in oligoastroastryomas/astrocytomas (30.7%) [140, 142, 144]. They occur in approximately 59-72% of OII and up to 64.2-100% of OIII and in 27-38% of OAII and 35.8-67% of OAIII [85, 140, 141, 145].

TERT promoter mutations are strongly associated with the classical oligodendroglial histology and co-occur with IDH1/2 mutations and 1p/19q co-deletion, suggesting a role in the oligodendroglial oncogenesis [134, 140, 141, 145, 146]. Moreover, they are associated with CIC mutations and EGFR gene amplification and are mutually exclusive with ATRX mutations [141, 146]. They have been found in approximately 66.7% of GBMO [144].

TERT mutations predict a favorable outcome in 1p/19q co-deleted tumors, whereas they are associated with a worse prognosis in tumors with intact 1p/19q and wild type IDH1/2 genes, similarly to GBMs [140]. When combined with the IDH1/2 status, they condition a better outcome and help identify prognostic subgroups of low- and high-grade gliomas [143–145].

By multivariate analysis, TERT mutations are independent prognostic markers for PFS and OS [140, 141, 145].

3.7. ATRX Mutations

The ATRX gene maps on chromosome Xq21.1 and encodes a protein that belongs to the H3.3 ATRX-DAXX chromatin-remodeling pathway [147]. ATRX is required for the binding of the histone variant H3.3 at pericentric chromatin and telomeres. ATRX perturbations may cause an alternative lengthening of telomeres (ALT) with genomic destabilization [148–150].

The ATRX mutation rate is in the range of 70% of IDH-mutant and 1p/19q intact low-grade gliomas [148, 150, 151]. Restricted to IDH-mutant tumors, they closely correlate with TP53 mutations and astrocytic differentiation and are mutually exclusive with 1p/19q co-deletion. ATRX mutations are typically observed in tumors of the so-called early progenitor-like transcriptional subclass (~85%), which has been linked to specific cells of origin in the forebrain SVZ to delineate the early progenitor-like low-grade gliomas [148, 151]. ATRX mutations occur in 47.8% of adult gliomas (37% truncated and 11.4% missense) and they are mainly localized in the highly conserved gene regions, especially in the helicase domain. Missense mutations may account for the discrepancy between molecular genetics and immunohistochemistry.

By the latter, positive nuclei denounce the absence of ATRX mutations in the tumor core (Figure 7E) and in infiltration areas or cortical satellitosis (Figure 7F, G). ATRX mutations and/or ATRX protein loss are significantly associated with the ALT phenotype [148, 150, 151].

Patients harboring ATRX mutations show a better outcome [150].

Although predominant in astrocytic tumors, ATRX mutations play the greatest role in the recognition of oligoastrocytomas [150]. In contrast to a mutation rate of 33-73% in anaplastic astrocytic tumors [151, 152, 153], they occur in 25% of OAII and in 27-53.8% of OAIII while they are absent or rare (<10%) in oligodendroglial tumors [150–153]. IHC revealed loss of ATRX protein expression in 27% of OAIII and in 7% of OIII [150]. Immunohistochemically, ATRX immunopositivity reveals the oligodendroglial component (Figure 7H).

In 43 cases, the absence of IDH1/2 mutations, 1p/19q co-deletion and the occurrence of TP53 and ATRX mutations have been found in astrocytic areas. Seventy *percent* of the cases were diagnosed as oligodendrogliomas due to the occurrence of astrocytes interpreted as reactive whereas the remaining 30% as astrocytomas. Oligoastrocytomas would no longer exist [76]. These results have been confirmed [77]. Contrary to this clear-cut position, other observations show that in mixed areas of oligoastrocytomas the results of ATRX IHC are heterogeneous in the astrocytic component and, therefore, the tumor still deserves the dignity of a tumor entity [154]. However, the non-existence of oligoastrocytomas was confirmed in a study of 152 astrocytomas, 61 oligodendrogliomas, 63 oligoastrocytomas and 129 GBMs where ATRX immunopositivity depicted endothelial cells, reactive astrocytes, microglia and lymphocytes [106]. Very importantly, it was observed that ATRX mutations do not occur in pilocytic astrocytomas [155].

Notably, ATRX mutations may be useful in identifying a subgroup of IDH-mutant astrocytic tumors with a favorable prognosis [150, 156].

3.8. CIC and FUBP1 Mutations

By high-throughput sequencing, recurrent somatic and inactivating mutations of CIC (homolog of the *Drosophila capicua gene*) and FUBP1 (Far Upstream Element [FUSE] Protein 1) genes have been identified in oligodendroglial tumors [107, 108, 109, 151, 157]. Both CIC and FUBP1 mutations would occur secondary to the unbalanced translocation, and their location on the chromosomal arms 1p (FUBP1) and 19q (CIC) support their putative roles as TSGs [107].

The CIC gene maps on the chromosomal region 19q13.2 and encodes a DNA-binding, high-mobility group (HMG)-box transcriptional repressor downstream of the receptor tyrosine kinase (RTK)-RAS-RAF-MAPK signaling pathways [158, 159]. CIC mutations occur in approximately 70% of 1p/19q co-deleted OIII and in only 7% of non-1p/19q co-deleted tumors. They are highly associated with the classical oligodendroglioma histology, 1p/19q co-deletion and IDH1/2 mutations [107, 109, 151]. The majority of CIC mutations (43%) cluster in exon 5 encoding the HMG-DNA binding domain and 58% of these are predicted to result in truncations of the encoded protein [107].

Associations have been reported with prognosis, PFS and OS [109]. CIC inactivating mutations may identify an aggressive subset of 1p19q co-deleted oligodendroglial tumors [160].

FUBP1 maps on the chromosomal region 1p31.1 and encodes a DNA helicase, which functions as transcriptional modulator of the c-Myc oncogene [161]. FUBP1 mutations have been identified in 15% of 1p/19q co-deleted and never in non-1p/19q co-deleted oligodendrogliomas. Interestingly, 75% of FUBP1 mutations occur in CIC-mutated oligodendrogliomas and are distributed within the FUPB1 DNA-binding site (encoded by exons 5–14) [107, 109]. They are rare (<10%) in OAII and OAIII [109, 151].

FUBP1 mutations may result in c-MYC activation and ribosome biogenesis.

In OII and OIII, FUBP1 mutations would not affect clinical outcome [162].

3.9. O^6-Methylguanine-DNA Methyltransferase (MGMT) Promoter Hypermethylation and G-CIMP

MGMT is a key DNA repair enzyme involved in the mechanism of resistance to alkylating agents. It specifically removes mutagenic, carcinogenic and cytotoxic O^6-alkylguanine DNA adducts induced by radiotherapy (RT) or alkylating agents as TMZ or nitrosourea derivatives. During malignant transformation, the MGMT gene may be epigenetically silenced by aberrant promoter hypermethylation, leading to an increased sensitivity to alkylating CHT with TMZ in malignant gliomas [163]. MGMT hypermethylation occurs in approximately 40% of gliomas with a higher rate in low than in high grade gliomas [164–167]. Among the former, it prevails in oligodendroglial tumors more than in mixed (50%) or astrocytic (31.9%) tumors [164–167].

MGMT promoter hypermethylation is strongly associated with IDH1/2 mutations and, thus, to the G-CIMP [168]. This finding may also partially explain the favorable clinical outcome of MGMT hypermethylated glioma patients after RT alone [169, 170]. Virtually, all 1p/19q co-deleted oligodendrogliomas show MGMT promoter hypermethylation and would belong to the G-CIMP [171]. Its prognostic role in grade III tumors is mainly related to IDH1/2 mutations, but it can be of benefit after alkylating CHT also in absence of IDH1/2 mutations [169, 170, 172]. In OIII, MGMT hypermethylation is the strongest predictive factor for CHT with procarbazine, lomustine (CCNU) and vincristine (PCV) [162, 173].

MGMT hypermethylation can be demonstrated immunohistochemically by the lack of MGMT protein expression in the nuclei of tumor cells (Figure 9A, B). IHC, however, is not sufficiently reliable to be indicated as a clinical biomarker for routine diagnostic purposes [174].

3.10. Epithelial Membrane Protein 3 (EMP3)

EMP3 is located on chromosome 19q13.3 and has been proposed as a candidate TSG for several malignancies, including gliomas [120, 128, 175, 176]. EMP3 encodes a myelin-related gene that belongs to the peripheral myelin protein 22-kDa (PMP22) gene family of small hydrophobic membrane glycoproteins [177]. It may be involved in cell proliferation, cell-cell interactions and apoptosis, and it would belong to the G-CIMP [168].

The EMP3 hypermethylation rate in low-grade gliomas is in the range of 63% in oligodendrogliomas and 70% in oligoastrocytomas [128, 176, 178]. In the former, it is strongly associated with IDH1/2 mutations and 1p/19q co-deletion but not with TP53 mutations or EGFR gene amplification.

Immunohistochemically, EMP3 aberrant hypermethylation may be revealed by the lack of EMP3 protein expression in the cytoplasms of tumor cells (Figure 9C, D).

EMP3 hypermethylation correlates with a better OS. At least, it can be proposed as a prognostic marker for oligodendroglial tumors [178].

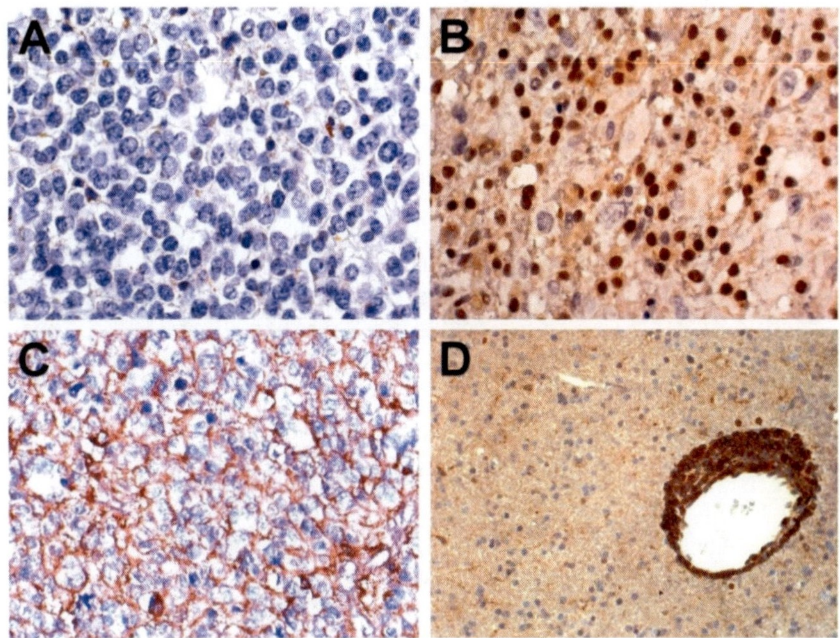

Figure 9. Anti-MGMT mouse monoclonal antibody (clone MT3.1, Chemicon International Inc., Temecula, CA, USA) immunohistochemistry (IHC): A – OII, Negative hypermethylated tumor cells, x400; B – OIII, positive unmethylated tumor cells, x400; Anti-EMP3 mouse monoclonal antibody (clone 3D4, Abnova, Taipei City, Taiwan) IHC: C – OIII, positive unmethylated tumor cells, x400. D – OIII, negative hypermethylated tumor cells and intensely positive perivascular cuffing of lymphocytes, x200. All DAB.

3.11. Anaplastic Oligodendroglioma

OIII has already been cited in the chapter, but here its discussion is resumed since it is important for prognosis and treatment. Compared to OII, OIII typically harbors additional genetic aberrations, including LOH on 9p21 and/or deletion of CDKN2A/B genes, EGFR gene amplification and polysomies [179, 180]. A homozygous deletion of the CDKN2A ($p16^{INK4A}$) gene is detectable in about one third of cases. This is more common in OIII with intact 1p/19q, although it may also be present in tumors with 1p/19q co-deletion. The adjacent CDKN2A ($p14^{ARF}$) and CDKN2B ($p15^{INK4B}$) genes are commonly deleted as well. A homozygous deletion of the CDKN2C gene and PTEN or PIK3CA mutations are restricted to <10% of OIII.

Polysomy on chromosome 7 and EGFR gene amplification prevail in OIII and OAIII more than grade II tumors, which are associated with TERT promoter mutations and implicate an unfavorable clinical outcome [179]. EGFR gene amplification, together with a homozygous deletion of the CDKN2A gene, is mutually exclusive with IDH1/2 mutations and 1p/19q co-deletion [181, 182].

Finally, polysomy of the chromosomal regions 1p and 19q predicts OIII shortened PFS [183] and unfavorable prognosis [184].

Recently, recurrent mutations in the TCF12 gene have been described in 7.5% of OIII [185]. Notably, TCF12 encodes an oligodendrocyte-related transcription factor. Eighty *percent* of all identified TCF12 mutations are located in the bHLH domain, critical for the TCF12 transcription function, or are frameshift mutations leading to a truncated protein. Mutations compromise TCF12 transcriptional activity, modify the subcellular protein localization and confer a more aggressive tumor phenotype. Moreover, TCF12 is highly expressed in neuronal progenitor cells during neuronal development [186] and in cells of the oligodendroglial lineage [187].

3.12. Pediatric Oligodendroglioma

The most striking difference with oligodendroglial tumors in adults is the absence of both 1p/19q co-deletion and IDH1/2 mutations [131, 188–190]. Tumors that harbor both genetic alterations usually occur in adolescents. This is in line with the rule that pediatric tumors resembling those of the adult are genetically different [191, 192].

Gains of function of the BRAF gene, by duplication or fusion to the KIAA1549 gene, have occasionally been reported in diffuse gliomas, more commonly oligodendroglial tumors [193 –195]. Recently, a BRAF-KIAA1549 fusion gene and deletion on the chromosomal arm 1p have been described in one case of oligodendroglioma with leptomeningeal dissemination [196].

3.13. GBMO

GBMO is a clinically and molecularly heterogeneous subgroup, predominantly classified into the Proneuronal and Classic GBM subtype in the EORTC 26981/NCIC CE.3 trial [51].

According to the IDH1/2 status, GBMO may be classified into two categories: with a higher IDH1/2 mutation rate, as in secondary GBMs, higher MGMT hypermethylation rate and lower frequency of EGFR gene amplification, and with lower IDH1/2 mutation rate, as in primary GBMs [197]. GBMO frequently shows 1p/19q co-deletion as well and, less commonly, LOH on the chromosomal arms 9p21 and 10q, irrespective of the IDH1/2 status [198–200]. Notably, IDH1/2 mutations have been proposed as a key step in the tumorigenesis of GBMO [201].

In contrast to adult patients, pediatric GBMO is characterized by an aggressive clinical phenotype, lack of IDH1/2 mutations and 1p/19q co-deletion, and by frequent microsatellite instability as a putative mechanism of TMZ resistance [202]. The different mutation rates in pediatric and adult tumors would support GBMO as a separate tumor entity with a different genetic background compared to pure oligodendroglial tumors [197].

The survival rate of GBMO patients is worse in comparison with OAIII without necrosis, but not significantly better compared to GBM patients [197, 200, 203]. GBMO OS is independent of the dominant histologic subtype, i.e., astrocytic or oligodendroglial, but it is significantly associated with the IDH1/2 status and with the MGMT hypermethylation status [197].

3.14. Timing and Relationships with Gliomagenesis

The discovery of the mutational landscape in oligodendrogliomas confirmed a mutually exclusive mutational profile in IDH mutated-1p/19q co-deleted and IDH mutated non-1p/19q co-deleted tumor subtypes. This corresponds to distinct molecular mechanisms of tumorigenesis that would implicate the subsequent acquisition of either the 1p/19q co-deletion and TERT promoter mutations or TP53 and ATRX mutations after IDH1/2 mutations (Figure 10) [143].

The common mechanism of tumor initiation in IDH mutated-1p/19q co-deleted would implicate IDH1/2 mutations as the earliest genetic event (driver mutation) preceding the 1p/19q co-deletion and TERT promoter mutation. This would predispose to a deactivation of CIC, FUBP1 and NOTCH genes and to activating mutations or gene amplifications in the PI3K pathway, and, histologically, to the classical oligodendroglioma phenotype. In contrast, the subsequent development of TP53 and ATRX mutations would predispose to the astrocytic phenotype [204–206].

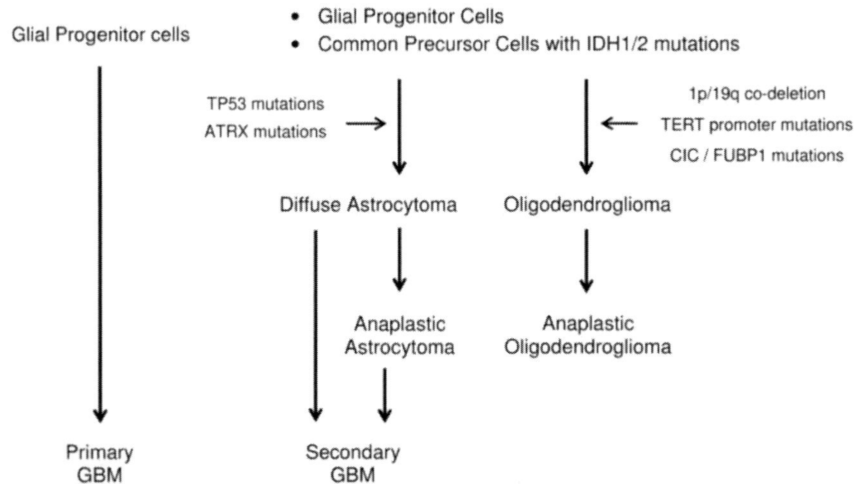

Figure 10. Model for the development of astrocytic and oligodendroglial tumors. Secondary glioblastomas (GBMs) (10%) develop from low-grade astrocytomas. Almost all cases harbor an IDH1/2 mutation and most of them also harbor TP53 and/or ATRX mutations. Primary GBMs (90%) arise *de novo* without IDH1/2 or ATRX mutations. Oligodendroglial tumors harbor an IDH1/2 mutation, 1p/19q co-deletion, TERT promoter mutations, CIC and FUBP1 mutations and wild type ATRX.

Together with IDH1/2 mutations, MGMT promoter hypermethylation is also an early epigenetic event during gliomagenesis of both astrocytic and oligodendrocytic tumors that precedes the differentiation of precursors [204, 207].

With regard to recurrences of low grade gliomas, at least half of the mutations detected in the primary tumor are not present at recurrence, including driver mutations such as TP53, ATRX, SMARCA4 and BRAF mutations [18]. This finding suggests that recurrence may be seeded by cells derived from the primary tumor at a very early stage of their evolution [18].

4. MicroRNAs (miRNAs)

Micro RNAs are small non-coding RNA molecules, approximately 21-25 nucleotides in length that post-transcriptionally regulate gene expression by translational inhibition or destabilization of the mRNA transcript. More than 1,500 precursors and 1,921 mature *Homo sapiens* miRNAs have been identified and reported in the miRBase database (Release 21, June 2014, http://www.mirbase.org/) [208]. A deregulation of miRNAs in oligodendroglial tumors has been suggested by several reports.

A comparative study between ten oligodendrogliomas and non-neoplastic samples identified several miRNAs up- (let-7a, let-7f, miR-17, miR-21, miR-155, miR-17, miR-16, miR-26b, miR-374a, let-7d, miR-20a, miR-15b, miR-7b, miR-9) or down-regulated (miR-132, miR-134, miR-7, miR-330-3p, miR-127-3p) [209]. Moreover, in the same study, a subset of seven markers (miR-21, miR-128, miR-132, miR-134, miR-155, miR-210 and miR-409-5p) was proposed as useful for differential diagnosis between oligodendroglial tumors and GBMs.

Interestingly, miR-9 is highly expressed in oligodendroglioma and the fetal brain, but at low levels in the adult brain, suggesting that miR-9 up-regulation may be important in the development of oligodendroglioma [210].

A comparison between newly-diagnosed OIII and recurrent tumors showed that seven miRNAs (miR-124, miR-128, miR-139-5p, miR-153, miR-210, miR-582-5p and miR-96) are highly increased in patients with recurrent anaplastic oligodendrogliomas. In particular, 5 miRNAs (miR-124, miR-128, miR-139-5p, miR-210 and miR-582-5p) exhibited more than 10-fold increased expression [211]. In contrast, 21 miRNAs (miR-1, miR-1180, miR-133b, miR-135b, miR-1539, miR-193a-5p, miR-196a, miR-196b, miR-200b, miR-21*, miR-221*, miR-224, miR-24-1*, miR-31, miR-31*, miR-32*, miR-34a*, miR-34c-5p, miR-455-5p, miR-503 and miR-631) showed a huge (0.01-fold) decreased expression in patients with recurrent OIII, if compared to those with newly-diagnosed tumors [211].

Finally, miR-137, which inhibits growth and invasion of glioma cells, was observed down-regulated in oligodendrogliomas and associated with shorter PFS and OS [212].

A recent study explored radiation-associated up or downregulation of miRNAs in OIII by comparing miRNA expression profiles in newly-diagnosed OIII to recurrent OIII treated with postoperative RT [211]. MiR-124, miR-128, miR-139-5p, miR-153, miR-210, miR-582-5p and miR-96 were highly increased in patients with recurrent OIII compared with newly-diagnosed OIII. In contrast, miR-1, miR-1180, miR-133b, miR-135b, miR-1539, miR-193a-5p, miR-196a, miR-196b, miR-200b, miR-21*, miR-221*, miR-224, miR-24-1*, miR-31, miR-32*, miR-34a*, miR-34c-5p, miR-455-5p, miR-503, and miR-631 showed extremely decreased expression in patients with recurrent OIII.

These are meaningful data for miRNAs as molecular tools for diagnosis and novel therapeutic targets in recurrent OIII treated with RT.

5. Treatment

The median survival time of OII ranges from 3.5 to 16.7 years [213, 214]. The median 5-year survival rate ranges from 38% to 83% [215, 216]. Oligodendrogliomas progress from grade II to grade III less frequently compared to astrocytomas [2]. The median post-surgical survival time of OIII ranges from 0.9 to 7.3 years [213, 217] with a median 5-year survival rate from 23% to 66% [84, 213, 217].

After surgery, OII can be followed according to the "wait and see" procedure or they can undergo RT with or without associated CHT, performed either immediately or after the "wait and see" procedure. In OII, RT prolongs the PFS of two years, but it does not affect OS [218]. The tumors respond to PCV, but only temporarily. OIII after surgery needs RT with adjuvant or post-radiation CHT, usually with PCV. The latter has been shown to be efficacious in GBMs [219, 220, 221], AIII [222], OIII [222, 223] and AII or OII [223–225].

Two phase III clinical trials (RTOG 9402 and EORTC 26951) recently demonstrated the favorable effects of combined RT and CHT with PCV in patients with OIII and OAIII with 1p/19q co-deletion. In the PCV-*plus*-RT arm, a median OS of 42 months *versus* 31 months in the RT-alone arm was observed, representing an improvement of 11 months in the entire intent-to-treat population. In patients harboring the 1p/19q co-deletion, the benefits were increased either with RT alone or in association with PCV (median OS has not yet been reached in the PCV-*plus*-RT arm whereas it was 112 months in the RT-alone arm) [50, 226].

TMZ is also used in the post-surgical treatment of oligodendrogliomas. In OIII, CHT prolongs the median time to progression to 25 months for responders [84, 227] and CHT *plus* RT up to 48 months [217].

Few reports are available on OA and GBMO. The median post-surgical survival time for OAII ranges from 3.9 to 5.3 years with a median 5-year survival rate of 58% [228]. OS of OAIII approximately corresponds to the value of AIII and it is shorter compared to OIII [229].

GBMO patients have a median post-surgical survival time of 19-26 months, a median PFS of 10.3 months and a median 2-year survival rate of 60%. Compared to GBMs, GBMO has a longer OS, but it affects patients of younger age. By comparing short-term survivors among GBMO patients (GBMO-STS) (survival $\leq$ 12 months) with long-term GBMO patients (GBMO-LTS) (survival $\geq$ 12 months), the former show the most dismal prognosis compared to OAIII, GBMO-LTS or GBMs [230].

6. PROGNOSIS

Different molecular markers have been identified as prognostic factors. In particular, 1p/19q co-deletion, IDH1/2 mutations and MGMT promoter hypermethylation, especially when associated with TMZ treatment, are strong prognostic markers in OII but scarcely in OIII [231, 232].

The assessment of the 1p/19q status is now commonly performed in patients with oligodendroglioma due to its significant prognostic and therapeutic implications. The long term follow up of two phase III clinical trials, The Radiation Therapy Oncology Group (RTOG) 9402 and The European Organization for Research and Treatment of Cancer (EORTC) 26951, have established the 1p/19q co-deletion as a prognostic and predictive marker of response to PCV regimen in OIII and OAIII patients [50, 226]. To date, this finding conditions the routine medical management of OIII patients with 1p/19q co-deletion (i.e., RT *plus* neoadjuvant or adjuvant PCV) [233–235]. Two further studies proved the predictive significance of the 1p/19q co-deletion also in response to TMZ regimen in both OIII and OAIII patients [236, 237]. Moreover, the results of the RTOG 9402 and EORTC 26591 studies proved a positive effect of the combined oncological treatment on PFS even among OIII and OAIII patients with intact 1p/19q [50, 226], also when TMZ is used [238].

With regard to IDH1/2 mutations, they are a significant marker of positive prognosis and chemosensitivity in low-grade gliomas when treated up-front with TMZ [80, 239]. In particular, patients with concurrent IDH1/2 mutations and 1p/19q co-deletion have the best prognosis [105]. Notably, in the RTOG 9402 clinical trial on adjuvant CHT with PCV in OIII, the IDH1/2 status emerged as a strong predictive factor of response to PCV [240].

MGMT promoter hypermethylation was initially discovered as a significant prognostic and predictive marker in patients with GBMs when treated with TMZ [163]. In oligodendrogliomas, MGMT hypermethylation is a positive prognostic marker, not predictive, when patients are treated with PCV, as proved by the EORTC 26951 and NOA-04 phase III clinical trials [169, 270]. In OIII patients treated with TMZ, MGMT hypermethylation showed only a borderline association with TMZ [236]. Remarkably, together with EMP3, MGMT belongs to the G-CIMP, recently described by the EORTC study 26951 as a better predictor of survival in comparison to MGMT hypermethylation in OIII patients [241].

LOH of 17p13, TP53 mutations and LOH on the chromosomal regions 10p and 10q, typically inversely correlated with the 1p/19q co-deletion, have a reduced prognostic significance in oligodendroglial tumors [24]. EGFR gene amplification, although rare in these tumors, conditions a reduced PFS in OIII [242]. In OIII patients with intact 1p/19q, EGFR gene amplification is associated with a poor prognosis [243]. The homozygous deletion of the CDKN2A ($p14^{ARF}$) gene on 9p21, prevalent in OIII, has been found to reduce OS [244–246], as well as LOH on chromosome 10q [247].

CONCLUSION

Recent high-throughput sequencing technologies have identified recurrent driver mutations in IDH1/2, TERT, CIC and FUBP1 mutations in oligodendroglial tumors, and, lastly, TCF12 mutations in OIII. The mutational landscape in oligodendrogliomas revealed a mutually exclusive mutational profile between IDH mutated-1p/19q co-deleted and IDH mutated non-1p/19q co-deleted tumor subtypes.

New molecular insights propose to incorporate molecular genetics analysis in the classical histologic diagnosis since they are instrumental to the clinical management of oligodendroglial tumors. In particular, a molecular classification based on the IDH1/2 and TERT mutational status and 1p/19q chromosomal status, together with ATRX, allows stratification of OII and OIII in well-defined clinically and morphological subgroups with important clinical implications.

A transition from a purely morphologic to an integrated morphologic and molecular classification of the heterogeneous group of the oligodendroglial tumors may result in improved management in terms of prognosis and therapy.

ACKNOWLEDGMENT

We thank Dr. M.C. Valentini (Neuroradiology Department/Città della Salute e della Scienza Hospital, Turin, Italy) for providing the MRI figures.

Disclosure of potential conflicts of interest: Authors declare no potential conflicts of interest.

REFERENCES

[1] Bailey, P; Bucy, P. Oligodendrogliomas of the brain. *The Journal of Pathology and Bacteriology*, 1929, 32, 735-754.

[2] Louis, DN; Ohgaki, H; Wiestler, OD; Cavenee, WK. *WHO Classification of Tumours of the Central Nervous System* (4th edition). Lyon, France: International Agency for Research on Cancer (IARC), 2007.

[3] Raff, MC; Miller, RH; Noble, M. A glial progenitor cell that develops *in vitro* into an astrocyte or an oligodendrocyte depending on culture medium. *Nature*, 1983, 303, 390-396.

[4] Liu, C; Sage, JC; Miller, MR; Verhaak, RG; Hippenmeyer, S; Vogel, H; Foreman, O; Bronson, RT; Nishiyama, A; Luo, L; Zong, H. Mosaic analysis with double markers reveals tumor cell of origin in glioma. *Cell*, 2011, 146, 209-221.

[5] Lindberg, N; Kastemar, M; Olofsson, T; Smits, A; Uhrbom, L. Oligodendrocyte progenitor cells can act as cell of origin for experimental glioma. *Oncogene*, 2009, 28, 2266-2275.

[6] Persson, AI; Petritsch, C; Swartling, FJ; Itsara, M; Sim, FJ; Auvergne, R; Goldenberg, DD; Vandenberg, SR; Nguyen, KN; Yakovenko, S; Ayers-Ringler, J; Nishiyama, A; Stallcup, WB; Berger, MS; Bergers, G; McKnight, TR; Goldman, SA; Weiss, WA. Non-stem cell origin for oligodendroglioma. *Cancer Cell*, 2010, 18, 669-682.

[7] Schiffer, D; Annovazzi, L; Caldera, V; Mellai, M. On the origin and growth of gliomas. *Anticancer Research*, 2010, 30, 1997-1998.

[8] Jiang, Y; Uhrbom, L. On the origin of glioma. *Upsala Journal of Medical Sciences*, 2012, 117, 113-121.

[9] Dawson, MR; Polito, A; Levine, JM; Reynolds, R. NG2-expressing glial progenitor cells: an abundant and widespread population of cycling cells in the adult rat CNS. *Molecular and Cellular Neurosciences*, 2003, 24, 476-488.

[10] Wilson, HC; Scolding, NJ; Raine, CS. Co-expression of PDGF alpha receptor and NG2 by oligodendrocyte precursors in human CNS and multiple sclerosis lesions. *Journal of Neuroimmunology*, 2006, 176, 162-173.

[11] Baracskay, KL; Kidd, GJ; Miller, RH; Trapp, BD. NG2-positive cells generate A2B5-positive oligodendrocyte precursor cells. *Glia*, 2007, 55, 1001-1010.

[12] Scherer, SS; Braun, PE; Grinspan, J; Collarini, E; Wang, DY; Kamholz, J. Differential regulation of the 2',3'-cyclic nucleotide 3'-phosphodiesterase gene during oligodendrocyte development. *Neuron*, 1994, 12, 1363-1375.

[13] Fruttiger, M; Karlsson, L; Hall, AC; Abramsson, A; Calver, AR; Boström, H; Willetts, K; Bertold, CH; Heath, JK; Betsholtz, C; Richardson, WD. Defective oligodendrocyte development and severe hypomyelination in PDGF-A knockout mice. *Development*, 1999, 126, 457-467.

[14] Cancer Genome Atlas Research Network. Comprehensive genomic characterization defines human glioblastoma genes and core pathways. *Nature*, 2008, 455, 1061-1068.

[15] Kondo, T; Raff, M. Oligodendrocyte precursor cells reprogrammed to become multipotential CNS stem cells. *Science*, 2000, 289, 1754-1757.

[16] Holland, EC; Celestino, J; Dai, C; Schaefer, L; Sawaya, RE; Fuller, GN. Combined activation of Ras and Akt in neural progenitors induces glioblastoma formation in mice. *Nature Genetics*, 2000, 25, 55-57.

[17] Holland, EC; Varmus, HE. Basic fibroblast growth factor induces cell migration and proliferation after glia-specific gene transfer in mice. *Proceedings of the National Academy of Sciences of the United States of America*, 1998, 95, 1218-1223.

[18] Johnson, BE; Mazor, T; Hong, C; Barnes, M; Aihara, K; McLean, CY; Fouse, SD; Yamamoto, S; Ueda, H; Tatsuno, K; Asthana, S; Jalbert, LE; Nelson, SJ; Bollen, AW; Gustafson, WC; Charron, E; Weiss, WA; Smirnov, IV; Song, JS; Olshen, AB; Cha, S; Zhao, Y; Moore, RA; Mungall, AJ; Jones, SJ; Hirst, M; Marra, MA; Saito, N; Aburatani, H; Mukasa, A; Berger, MS; Chang, SM; Taylor, BS; Costello, JF. Mutational analysis reveals the origin and therapy-driven evolution of recurrent glioma. *Science*, 2014, 343, 189-193.

[19] Ostrom, QT; Bauchet, L; Davis, FG; Deltour, I; Fisher, JL; Langer, CE; Pekmezci, M; Schwartzbaum, JA; Turner, MC; Walsh, KM; Wrensch, MR; Barnholtz-Sloan, JS. The epidemiology of glioma in adults: a "state of the science" review. *Neuro Oncology*, 2014, 16, 896-913.

[20] Mørk, SJ; Halvorsen, TB; Lindegaard, KF; Eide, GE. Oligodendroglioma. Histologic evaluation and prognosis. *Journal of Neuropathology and Experimental Neurology*, 1986, 45, 65-78.

[21] Ludwig, CL; Smith, MT; Godfrey, AD; Armbrustmacher, VW. A clinicopathological study of 323 patients with oligodendrogliomas. *Annals of Neurology*, 1986, 19, 15-21.

[22] Reifenberger, G; Kros, JM; Louis, DM; Collins, VP. Oligodendroglioma. In: Louis, DN; Ohgaki, H; Wiestler, OD; Cavenee, WK, Eds. *WHO Classification of Tumours of the Central Nervous System* (4th edition). Lyon, France: International Agency for Research on Cancer (IARC), 2007, 54-59.

[23] Von Deimling, A; Reifenberger G; Kros, JM; Louis, DN; Collins, VP. Oligoatrocytoma. In: Louis, DN; Ohgaki, H; Wiestler, OD; Cavenee, WK, Eds. *WHO Classification of Tumours of the Central Nervous System* (4th edition). Lyon, France: International Agency for Research on Cancer (IARC), 2007, 63-65.

[24] Von Deimling, A. *Gliomas*. Berlin Heidelberg, Germany: Springer-Verlag, 2009.

[25] Schiffer, D. *Brain Tumors. Biology, Pathology, and Clinical References*. 2th edition. Berlin Heidelberg, Germany: Springer-Verlag, 1993, 1997.

[26] Reiche, W; Grunwald, I; Hermann, K; Deinzer, M; Reith, W. Oligodendrogliomas. *Acta Radiologica*, 2002, 43, 474-482.

[27] White, ML; Zhang, Y; Kirby, P; Ryken, TC. Can tumor contrast enhancement be used as a criterion for differentiating tumor grades of oligodendrogliomas? *AJNR. American Journal of Neuroradiology*, 2005, 26, 784-790.

[28] Khalid, L; Carone, M; Dumrongpisutikul, N; Intrapiromkul, J; Bonekamp, D; Barker, PB; Yousem, DM. Imaging characteristics of oligodendrogliomas that predict grade. *AJNR. American Journal of Neuroradiology*, 2012, 33, 852-857.

[29] Kono, K; Inoue, Y; Nakayama, K; Shakudo, M; Morino, M; Ohata, K; Wakasa, K; Yamada, R. The role of diffusion-weighted imaging in patients with brain tumors. *AJNR. American Journal of Neuroradiology*, 2001, 22, 1081-1088.

[30] Whitmore, RG; Krejza, J; Kapoor, GS; Huse, J; Woo, JH; Bloom, S; Lopinto, J; Wolf, RL; Judy, K; Rosenfeld, MR; Biegel, JA; Melhem, ER; O'Rourke, DM. Prediction of oligodendroglial tumor subtype and grade using perfusion weighted magnetic resonance imaging. *Journal of Neurosurgery*, 2007, 107, 600-609.

[31] Spampinato, MV; Smith, JK; Kwock, L; Ewend, M; Grimme, JD; Camacho, DL; Castillo, M. Cerebral blood volume measurements and proton MR spectroscopy in grading of oligodendroglial tumors. *AJR. American Journal of Roentgenology*, 2007, 188, 204-212.

[32] Lev, MH; Ozsunar, Y; Henson, JW; Rasheed, AA; Barest, GD; Harsh, GR 4th; Fitzek, MM; Chiocca, EA; Rabinov, JD; Csavoy, AN; Rosen,

BR; Hochberg, FH; Schaefer, PW; Gonzalez, RG. Glial tumor grading and outcome prediction using dynamic spin-echo MR susceptibility mapping compared with conventional contrast-enhanced MR: confounding effect of elevated rCBV of oligodendrogliomas. *AJNR. American Journal of Neuroradiology*, 2004, 25, 214-221.

[33] Xu, M; See, SJ; Ng, WH; Arul, E; Back, MF; Yeo, TT; Lim, CC. Comparison of magnetic resonance spectroscopy and perfusion-weighted imaging in presurgical grading of oligodendroglial tumors. *Neurosurgery*, 2005, 56, 919-926.

[34] Koellner, KK; Rushsing, EJ. Oligodendroglioma and Its Variants: Radiologic-Pathologic Correlation. *RadioGraphics*, 2005, 25, 1669-1688.

[35] Schiffer, D; Dutto, A; Cavalla, P; Chiò, A; Migheli, A; Piva, R. Role of apoptosis in the prognosis of oligodendrogliomas. *Neurochemistry international*, 1997, 31, 245-250.

[36] Schiffer, D; Cravioto, H; Giordana, MT; Migheli, A; Pezzulo, T; Vigliani, MC. Is polar spongioblastoma a tumor entity? *Journal of Neurosurgery*, 1993 78, 587-591.

[37] Schiffer, D; Dutto, A; Cavalla, P; Bosone, I; Chiò, A; Villani, R; Bellotti, C. Prognostic factors in oligodendroglioma. *The Canadian Journal of Neurological Sciences*, 1997, 24, 313-319.

[38] Giannini, C; Scheithauer, BW; Weaver, AL; Burger, PC; Kros, JM; Mork, S; Graeber, MB; Bauserman, S; Buckner, JC; Burton, J; Riepe, R; Tazelaar, HD; Nascimento, AG; Crotty, T; Keeney, GL; Pernicone, P; Altermatt, H. Oligodendrogliomas: reproducibility and prognostic value of histologic diagnosis and grading. *Journal of Neuropathology and Experimental Neurology*, 2001, 60, 248-262.

[39] Kros, JM; Troost, D; van Eden, CG; van der Werf, AJ; Uylings, HB. Oligodendroglioma. A comparison of two grading systems. *Cancer*, 1988, 61, 2251-2259.

[40] Miller, Cr; Dunham, CP; Scheithauer, BW; Perry, A. Significance of necrosis in grading oligodendroglial neoplasms: a clinicopathologic and genetic study of newly diagnosed high-grade gliomas. *Journal of Clinical Oncology*, 2006, 24, 5419-5426.

[41] Donahue, B; Scott, CB; Nelson, JS; Rotman, M; Murray, KJ; Nelson, DF; Banker, FL; Earle, JD; Fischbach, JA; Asbell, SO; Gaspar, LE; Markoe, AM; Curran, W. Influence of an oligodendroglial component on the survival of patients with anaplastic astrocytomas: a report of

Radiation Therapy Oncology Group 83-02. *International Journal of Radiation Oncology, Biology, Physics*, 1997, 38, 911-914.

[42] De Armond, SJ; Eng, LF; Rubinstein, LJ. The application of glial fibrillary acidic (GFA) protein immunohistochemistry in neurooncology. A progress report. *Pathology, Research and Practice*, 1980, 168, 374-394.

[43] Van der Meulen, JD; Houthoff, HJ; Ebels, EJ. Glial fibrillary acidic protein in human gliomas. *Neuropathology and Applied Neurobiology*, 1978, 4, 177-190.

[44] Raff, MC. Glial cell diversification *Science*, 1989 243, 1450-1455.

[45] Herpers, MJ; Budka, H. Glial fibrillary acidic protein (GFAP) in oligodendroglial tumors: gliofibrillary oligodendroglioma and transitional oligoastrocytoma as subtypes of oligodendroglioma. *Acta Neuropathologica*, 1984, 64, 265-272.

[46] Choi, BH; Kim, RC. Expression of glial fibrillary acidic protein in immature oligodendroglia. *Science*, 1984, 223, 407-409.

[47] Schiffer, D. *Brain Tumor Pathology: Current Diagnostic Hotspots and Pitfalls*. Dordrecht, Netherlands: Springer; 2006.

[48] Coons, SW; Johnson, PC; Pearl, DK. The prognostic significance of Ki-67 labeling indices for oligodendrogliomas. *Neurosurgery*, 1997, 41, 878-884.

[49] Krouwer, HG; Van Duinen, SG; Kamphorst, W; van der Valk, P; Algra, A. Oligoastrocytomas: a clinicopathological study of 52 cases. *Journal of NeuroOncology*, 1997, 3, 223-238.

[50] van den Bent, MJ; Carpentier, AF; Brandes, AA; Sanson, M; Taphoorn, MJ; Bernsen, HJ; Frenay, M; Tijssen, CC; Grisold, W; Sipos, L; Haaxma-Reiche, H; Kros, JM; van Kouwenhoven, MC; Vecht, CJ; Allgeier, A; Lacombe, D; Gorlia T. Adjuvant procarbazine, lomustine, and vincristine improves progression-free survival but not overall survival in newly diagnosed anaplastic oligodendrogliomas and oligoastrocytomas: a randomized European Organisation for Research and Treatment of Cancer phase III trial. *Journal of Clinical Oncology*, 2006, 24, 2715-2722.

[51] Hegi, ME; Janzer, RC; Lambiv, WL; Gorlia, T; Kouwenhoven, MC; Hartmann, C; von Deimling, A; Martinet, D; Besuchet Schmutz, N; Diserens, AC; Hamou, MF; Bady, P; Weller, M; van den Bent, MJ; Mason, WP; Mirimanoff, RO; Stupp, R; Mokhtari, K; Wesseling, P; European Organisation for Research and Treatment of Cancer Brain Tumour and Radiation Oncology Groups; National Cancer Institute of

Canada Clinical Trials Group. Presence of an oligodendroglioma-like component in newly diagnosed glioblastoma identifies a pathogenetically heterogeneous subgroup and lacks prognostic value: central pathology review of the EORTC_26981/NCIC_CE.3 trial. *Acta Neuropathologica*, 2012, 123, 841-852.

[52] Ha, SY; Kang, SY; Do, IG; Suh, YL. Glioblastoma with oligodendroglial component represents a subgroup of glioblastoma with high prevalence of IDH1 mutation and association with younger age. *Journal of NeuroOncology*, 2013, 112, 439-448.

[53] Nishie, A; Ono, M; Shono, T; Fukushi, J; Otsubo, M; Onoue, H; Ito, Y; Inamura, T; Ikezaki, K; Fukui, M; Iwaki, T; Kuwano, M. Macrophage infiltration and heme oxygenase-1 expression correlate with angiogenesis in human gliomas. *Clinical Cancer Research*, 1999, 5, 1107-1113.

[54] Nishie, A; Masuda, K; Otsubo, M; Migita, T; Tsuneyoshi, M; Kohno, K; Shuin, T; Naito, S; Ono, M; Kuwano, M. High expression of the Cap43 gene in infiltrating macrophages of human renal cell carcinomas. *Clinical Cancer Research*, 2001, 7, 2145-2151.

[55] Deininger, MH; Weller, M; Streffer, J; Mittelbronn, M; Meyermann, R. MPattern of cyclooxygenase-1 and -2 expression in human gliomas *in vivo*. *Acta Neuropathologica*, 1999, 98, 240-244.

[56] Deininger, MH; Meyermann, R; Trautmann, K; Duffner, F; Grote, EH; Wickboldt, J; Schluesener, HJ. Heme oxygenase (HO)-1 expressing macrophages/microglial cells accumulate during oligodendroglioma progression. *Brain Research*, 2000, 882, 1-8.

[57] Sasaki, A; Yokoo, H; Tanaka, Y; Homma, T; Nakazato, Y; Ohgaki, H. Characterization of microglia/macrophages in gliomas developed in S-100β-v-erbB transgenic rats. *Neuropathology*, 2013, 33, 505-514.

[58] Kamper, P; Bendix, K; Hamilton-Dutoit, S; Honoré, B; Nyengaard, JR; D'Amore F. Tumor-infiltrating macrophages correlate with adverse prognosis and Epstein-Barr virus status in classical Hodgkin's lymphoma. *Haematologica*, 2011, 96, 269-276.

[59] Zaki, MA; Wada, N; Ikeda, J; Shibayama, H; Hashimoto, K; Yamagami, T; Tatsumi, Y; Tsukaguchi, M; Take, H; Tsudo, M; Morii, E; Aozasa, K. Prognostic implication of types of tumor-associated macrophages in Hodgkin lymphoma. *Virchows Archiv*, 2011, 459, 361-366.

[60] Ino, Y; Yamazaki-Itoh, R; Shimada, K; Iwasaki, M; Kosuge, T; Kanai, Y; Hiraoka, N. Immune cell infiltration as an indicator of the immune

microenvironment of pancreatic cancer. *British Journal of Cancer*, 2013, 108, 914-923.

[61] Herrera, M; Herrera, A; Domínguez, G; Silva, J; García, V; García, JM; Gómez, I; Soldevilla, B; Muñoz, C; Provencio, M; Campos-Martin, Y; García de Herreros, A; Casal, I; Bonilla, F; Peña, C. Cancer-associated fibroblast and M2 macrophage markers together predict outcome in colorectal cancer patients. *Cancer Science*, 2013, 104, 437-444.

[62] Barros, MH; Hauck, F; Dreyer, JH; Kempkes, B; Niedobitek, G. Macrophage polarisation: an immunohistochemical approach for identifying M1 and M2 macrophages. *PLoS One*, 2013, 8, e80908.

[63] Szulzewsky, F; Pelz, A; Feng, X; Synowitz, M; Markovic, D; Langmann, T; Holtman, IR; Wang, X; Eggen, BJ; Boddeke, HW; Hambardzumyan, D; Wolf, SA; Kettenmann, H. Glioma-associated microglia/macrophages display an expression profile different from M1 and M2 polarization and highly express Gpnmb and Spp1. *PLoS One*, 2015, 10, e0116644.

[64] Kennedy, BC; Showers, CR; Anderson, DE; Anderson, L; Canoll, P; Bruce, JN; Anderson, RC. Tumor-associated macrophages in glioma: friend or foe? *Journal of Oncology*, 2013, 2013, 486912.

[65] Decaestecker, C; Lopes, BS; Gordower, L; Camby, I; Cras, P; Martin, JJ; Kiss, R; VandenBerg, SR; Salmon, I. Quantitative chromatin pattern description in Feulgen-stained nuclei as a diagnostic tool to characterize the oligodendroglial and astroglial components in mixed oligo-astrocytomas. *Journal of Neuropathology and Experimental Neurology*. 1997, 56, 391-402.

[66] Burger, PC. What is an oligodendroglioma? *Brain Pathology*, 2002, 12, 257-259.

[67] Daumas-Duport, C; Varlet, P; Tucker, ML; Beuvon, F; Cervera, P; Chodkiewicz, JP. Oligodendrogliomas. Part I: Patterns of growth, histological diagnosis, clinical and imaging correlations: a study of 153 cases. *Journal of Neurooncology*, 1997, 34, 37-59.

[68] Fortin, D; Cairncross, GJ; Hammond, RR. Oligodendroglioma: an appraisal of recent data pertaining to diagnosis and treatment. *Neurosurgery*, 1999, 45, 1279-1291.

[69] Bosone, I; Cavalla, P; Chiadò-Piat, L; Vito, ND; Schiffer, D. Cyclin D1 expression in normal oligodendroglia and microglia cells: its use in the differential diagnosis of oligodendrogliomas. *Neuropathology*, 2001, 21, 155-161.

[70] Cavalla, P; Piva, R; Bortolotto, S; Grosso, R; Cancelli, I; Chiò, A; Schiffer, D. p27/kip1 expression in oligodendrogliomas and its possible prognostic role. *Acta Neuropathologica*, 1999, 98, 629-634.

[71] Bouvier, C; Bartoli, C; Aguirre-Cruz, L; Virard, I; Colin, C; Fernandez, C; Gouvernet, J; Figarella-Branger, D. Shared oligodendrocyte lineage gene expression in gliomas and oligodendrocyte progenitor cells. *Journal of Neurosurgery*, 2003, 99, 344-350.

[72] Riemenschneider, MJ; Koy, TH; Reifenberger, G. Expression of oligodendrocyte lineage genes in oligodendroglial and astrocytic gliomas. *Acta Neuropathologica*, 2004, 107, 277-282.

[73] Azzarelli, B; Miravalle, L; Vidal, R. Immunolocalization of the oligodendrocyte transcription factor 1 (Olig1) in brain tumors. *Journal of Neuropathology and Experimental Neurology*, 2004, 63, 170-179.

[74] Ligon, KL; Alberta, JA; Kho, AT; Weiss, J; Kwaan, MR; Nutt, CL; Louis, DN; Stiles, CD; Rowitch, DH. The oligodendroglial lineage marker OLIG2 is universally expressed in diffuse gliomas. *Journal of Neuropathology and Experimental Neurology*, 2004, 63, 499-509.

[75] Blümcke, I; Becker, AJ; Normann, S; Hans, V; Riederer, BM; Krajewski, S; Wiestler, OD; Reifenberger, G. Distinct expression pattern of microtubule-associated protein-2 in human oligodendrogliomas and glial precursor cells. *Journal of Neuropathology and Experimental Neurology*, 2001, 60, 984-993.

[76] Figarella-Branger, D; Mokhtari, K; Dehais, C; Jouvet, A; Uro-Coste, E; Colin, C; Carpentier, C; Forest, F; Maurage, CA; Vignaud, JM; Polivka, M; Lechapt-Zalcman, E; Eimer, S; Viennet, G; Quintin-Roué, I; Aubriot-Lorton, MH; Diebold, MD; Loussouarn, D; Lacroix, C; Rigau, V; Laquerrière, A; Vandenbos, F; Michalak, S; Sevestre, H; Peoch, M; Labrousse, F; Christov, C; Kemeny, JL; Chenard, MP; Chiforeanu, D; Ducray, F; Idbaih, A; POLA Network. Mitotic index, microvascular proliferation, and necrosis define 3 groups of 1p/19q codeleted anaplastic oligodendrogliomas associated with different genomic alterations. *Neuro-Oncology*, 2014, 16, 1244-1254.

[77] Sahm, F; Reuss, D; Koelsche, C; Capper, D; Schittenhelm, J; Heim, S; Jones, DT; Pfister, SM; Herold-Mende, C; Wick, W; Mueller, W; Hartmann, C; Paulus, W; von Deimling, A. Farewell to oligoastrocytoma: in situ molecular genetics favor classification as either oligodendroglioma or astrocytoma. *Acta Neuropathologica*, 2014, 128, 551-559.

[78] Appin, CL; Brat, DJ. Molecular genetics of gliomas. *Cancer Journal*, 2014, 20, 66-72.

[79] Wilcox, P; Li, CC; Lee, M; Shivalingam, B; Brennan, J; Suter, CM; Kaufman, K; Lum, T; Buckland, ME. Oligoastrocytomas: throwing the baby out with the bathwater? *Acta Neuropathologica*, 2015, 129, 147-149.

[80] Sanson, M; Marie, Y; Paris, S; Idbaih, A; Laffaire, J; Ducray, F; El Hallani, S; Boisselier, B; Mokhtari, K; Hoang-Xuan, K; Delattre, JY. Isocitrate dehydrogenase 1 codon 132 mutation is an important prognostic biomarker in gliomas. *Journal of Clinical Oncology,* 2009, 27, 4150-4154.

[81] Yan, H; Parsons, DW; Jin, G; McLendon, R; Rasheed, BA; Yuan, W; Kos, I; Batinic-Haberle, I; Jones, S; Riggins, GJ; Friedman, H; Friedman, A; Reardon, D; Herndon, J; Kinzler, KW; Velculescu, VE; Vogelstein, B; Bigner, DD. IDH1 and IDH2 mutations in gliomas. *The New England Journal of Medicine*, 2009, 360, 765-773.

[82] Hartmann, C; Meyer, J; Balss, J; Capper, D; Mueller, W; Christians, A; Felsberg, J; Wolter, M; Mawrin, C; Wick, W; Weller, M; Herold-Mende, C; Unterberg, A; Jeuken, JW; Wesseling, P; Reifenberger, G; von Deimling, A. Type and frequency of IDH1 and IDH2 mutations are related to astrocytic and oligodendroglial differentiation and age: a study of 1,010 diffuse gliomas. *Acta Neuropathologica*, 2009, 118, 469-474.

[83] Reifenberger, J; Reifenberger, G; Liu, L; James, CD; Wechsler, W; Collins, VP. Molecular genetic analysis of oligodendroglial tumors shows preferential allelic deletions on 19q and 1p. *The American Journal of Pathology*, 1994, 145, 1175-1190.

[84] Cairncross, JG; Ueki, K; Zlatescu, MC; Lisle, DK; Finkelstein, DM; Hammond, RR; Silver, JS; Stark, PC; Macdonald, DR; Ino, Y; Ramsay, DA; Louis, DN. Specific genetic predictors of chemotherapeutic response and survival in patients with anaplastic oligodendrogliomas. *Journal of the National Cancer Institute*, 1998, 90, 1473-1479.

[85] Eckel-Passow, JE; Lachance, DH; Molinaro, AM; Walsh, KM; Decker, PA; Sicotte, H; Pekmezci, M; Rice, T; Kosel, ML; Smirnov, IV; Sarkar, G; Caron, AA; Kollmeyer, TM; Praska, CE; Chada, AR; Halder, C; Hansen, HM; McCoy, LS; Bracci, PM; Marshall, R; Zheng, S; Reis, GF; Pico, AR; O'Neill, BP; Buckner, JC; Giannini, C; Huse, JT; Perry, A; Tihan, T; Berger, MS; Chang, SM; Prados, MD; Wiemels, J; Wiencke, JK; Wrensch, MR; Jenkins, RB. Glioma Groups Based on 1p/19q, IDH,

and TERT Promoter Mutations in Tumors. *New England Journal of Medicine.* 2015, 372, 2499-508.

[86] Thon, N; Eigenbrod, S; Kreth, S; Lutz, J; Tonn, JC; Kretzschmar, H; Peraud, A; Kreth, FW. IDH1 mutations in grade II astrocytomas are associated with unfavorable progression-free survival and prolonged postrecurrence survival. *Cancer*, 2012, 118, 452-460.

[87] Mueller, W; Hartmann, C; Hoffmann, A; Lanksch, W; Kiwit, J; Tonn, J; Veelken, J; Schramm, J; Weller, M; Wiestler, OD; Louis, DN; von Deimling, A. Genetic signature of oligoastrocytomas correlates with tumor location and denotes distinct molecular subsets. *The American Journal of Pathology*, 2002, 161, 313-319.

[88] Burger, PC; Minn, AY; Smith, JS; Borell, TJ; Jedlicka, AE; Huntley, BK; Goldthwaite, PT; Jenkins, RB; Feuerstein, BG. Losses of chromosomal arms 1p and 19q on the diagnosis of oligodendroglioma. Study of paraffin-embedded sections. *Modern Pathology*, 2001, 14, 842-853.

[89] McDonald, JM; See, SJ; Tremont, IW; Colman, H; Gilbert, MR; Groves, M; Burger, PC; Louis, DN; Giannini, C; Fuller, G; Passe, S; Blair, H; Jenkins, RB; Yang, H; Ledoux, A; Aaron, J; Tipnis, U; Zhang, W; Hess, K; Aldape, K. The prognostic impact of histology and 1p/19q status in anaplastic oligodendroglial tumors. *Cancer*, 2005, 104, 1468-1477.

[90] Wharton, SB; Hamilton, FA; Chan, WK; Chan, KK; Anderson, JR. Proliferation and cell death in oligodendrogliomas. *Neuropathology and Applied Neurobiology*, 2007, 24, 21-28.

[91] Schiffer, D; Cavalla, P; Migheli, A; Chiò, A; Giordana, MT; Marino, S; Attanasio, A. Apoptosis and cell proliferation in human neuroepithelial tumors. *Neuroscience Letters*, 1995, 195, 81-84.

[92] Reifenberger, G; Louis, DN. Oligodendroglioma. Toward molecular definition in diagnostic neurooncology. *Journal of Neuropathology and Experimental Neurology*, 2003, 62, 11-126.

[93] Kros, JM; van der Weiden, M; Zheng, PP; Hop, WC; van den Bent, MJ; Kouwenhoven, MC. Intratumoral distribution of 1p loss in oligodendroglial tumors. *Journal of Neuropathology and Experimental Neurology*, 2007, 66, 1118-1123.

[94] van Thuijl, HF; Scheinin, I; Sie, D; Alentorn, A; van Essen, HF; Cordes, M; Fleischeuer, R; Gijtenbeek, AM; Beute, G; van den Brink, WA; Meijer, GA; Havenith, M; Idbaih, A; Hoang-Xuan, K; Mokhtari, K; Verhaak, RG; van der Valk, P; van de Wiel, MA; Heimans, JJ; Aronica, E; Reijneveld, JC; Wesseling, P; Ylstra, B. Spatial and temporal

evolution of distal 10q deletion, a prognostically unfavorable event in diffuse low-grade gliomas. *Genome Biology*, 2014, 15, 471.

[95] Appin, CL; Gao, J; Chisolm, C; Torian, M; Alexis, D; Vincentelli, C; Schniederjan, MJ; Hadjipanayis, C; Olson, JJ; Hunter, S; Hao, C; Brat DJ. Glioblastoma *Brain Pathology*, 2013, 23, 454-461.

[96] He, J; Mokhtari, K; Sanson, M; Marie, Y; Kujas, M; Huguet, S; Leuraud, P; Capelle, L; Delattre, JY; Poirier, J; Hoang-Xuan, K. Glioblastomas with an oligodendroglial component: a pathological and molecular study. *Journal of Neuropathology and Experimental Neurology*, 2001, 60, 863-871.

[97] Rodriguez, FJ; Scheithauer, BW; Jenkins, R; Burger, PC; Rudzinskiy, P; Vlodavsky, E; Schooley, A; Landolfi, J. Gliosarcoma arising in oligodendroglial tumors ("oligosarcoma"): a clinicopathologic study. *The American Journal of Surgical Pathology*, 2007, 31, 351-362.

[98] Griffin, CA; Burger, P; Morsberger, L; Yonescu, R; Swierczynski, S; Weingart, JD; Murphy, KM. Identification of der(1;19)(q10;p10) in five oligodendrogliomas suggests mechanism of concurrent 1p and 19q loss. *Journal of Neuropathology and Experimental Neurology*, 2006, 65, 988-994.

[99] Jenkins, RB; Blair, H; Ballman, KV; Giannini, C; Arusell, RM; Law, M; Flynn, H; Passe, S; Felten, S; Brown, PD; Shaw, EG; Buckner, JC. A t(1;19)(q10;p10) mediates the combined deletions of 1p and 19q and predicts a better prognosis of patients with oligodendroglioma. *Cancer Research*, 2006, 66, 9852-9861.

[100] Gadji, M; Tsanaclis, A-M; Fortin, D; Drouin, R. Aneuploidy and chromosomal instability in gliomas. *Proceedings of the 99th Annual Meeting of the American Association for Cancer Research (AACR), Philadelphia, PA*, 2008, Ab nr 4331.

[101] Idbaih, A; Marie, Y; Pierron, G; Brennetot, C; Hoang-Xuan, K; Kujas, M; Mokhtari, K; Sanson, M; Lejeune, J; Aurias, A; Delattre, O; Delattre, JY. Two types of chromosome 1p losses with opposite significance in gliomas. *Annals of Neurology,* 2005, 58, 483-487.

[102] Barbashina, V; Salazar, P; Holland, EC; Rosenblum, MK; Ladanyi, M. *Clinical Cancer Research,* 2005, 11, 1119-1128.

[103] Hartmann, C; Johnk, L; Kitange, G; Wu, Y; Ashworth, LK; Jenkins, RB; Louis, DN. Transcript map of the 3.7-Mb D19S112-D19S246 candidate tumor suppressor region on the long arm of chromosome 19. *Cancer Research*, 2002, 62, 4100-4108.

[104] von Deimling, A; Bender, B; Jahnke, R; Waha, A; Kraus, J; Albrecht, S; Wellenreuther, R; Fassbender, F; Nagel, J; Menon, AG, et al. Loci associated with malignant progression in astrocytomas: a candidate on chromosome 19q. *Cancer Research*, 1994, 54, 1397-1401.

[105] Labussière, M; Idbaih, A; Wang, XW; Marie, Y; Boisselier, B; Falet, C; Paris, S; Laffaire, J; Carpentier, C; Crinière, E; Ducray, F; El Hallani, S; Mokhtari, K; Hoang-Xuan, K; Delattre, JY; Sanson, M. All the 1p19q codeleted gliomas are mutated on IDH1 or IDH2. *Neurology*, 2010, 74, 1886-1890.

[106] Reuss, DE; Sahm, F; Schrimpf, D; Wiestler, B; Capper, D; Koelsche, C; Schweizer, L; Korshunov, A; Jones, DT; Hovestadt, V; Mittelbronn, M; Schittenhelm, J; Herold-Mende, C; Unterberg, A; Platten, M; Weller, M; Wick, W; Pfister, SM; Von Deimling, A. ATRX and IDH1-R132H immunohistochemistry with subsequent copy number analysis and IDH sequencing as a basis for an "integrated" diagnostic approach for adult astrocytoma, oligodendroglioma and glioblastoma. *Acta Neuropathologica*, 2015, 129, 133-146.

[107] Bettegowda, C; Agrawal, N; Jiao, Y; Sausen, M; Wood, LD; Hruban, RH; Rodriguez, FJ; Cahill, DP; McLendon, R; Riggins, G; Velculescu, VE; Oba-Shinjo, SM; Marie, SK; Vogelstein, B; Bigner, D; Yan, H; Papadopoulos, N; Kinzler, KW. Mutations in CIC and FUBP1 contribute to human oligodendroglioma. *Science*, 2011, 333, 1453-1455.

[108] Yip, S; Butterfield, YS; Morozova, O; Chittaranjan, S; Blough, MD; An, J; Birol, I; Chesnelong, C; Chiu, R; Chuah, E; Corbett, R; Docking, R; Firme, M; Hirst, M; Jackman, S; Karsan, A; Li, H; Louis, DN; Maslova, A; Moore, R; Moradian, A; Mungall, KL; Perizzolo, M; Qian, J; Roldan, G; Smith, EE; Tamura-Wells, J; Thiessen, N; Varhol, R; Weiss, S; Wu, W; Young, S; Zhao, Y; Mungall, AJ; Jones, SJ; Morin, GB; Chan, JA; Cairncross, JG; Marra, MA. Concurrent CIC mutations, IDH mutations, and 1p/19q loss distinguish oligodendrogliomas from other cancers. *The Journal of Pathology*, 2012, 226, 7-16.

[109] Sahm, F; Koelsche, C; Meyer, J; Pusch, S; Lindenberg, K; Mueller, W; Herold-Mende, C; von Deimling, A; Hartmann, C. CIC and FUBP1 mutations in oligodendrogliomas, oligoastrocytomas and astrocytomas. *Acta Neuropathologica*, 2012, 123, 853-860.

[110] Ducray, F; Idbaih, A; de Reyniès, A; Bièche, I; Thillet, J; Mokhtari, K; Lair, S; Marie, Y; Paris, S; Vidaud, M; Hoang-Xuan, K; Delattre, O; Delattre, JY; Sanson, M. Anaplastic oligodendrogliomas with 1p19q

codeletion have a proneural gene expression profile. *Molecular Cancer*, 2008, 20, 7-41.

[111] Ichimura, K; Vogazianou, AP; Liu, L; Pearson, DM; Bäcklund, LM; Plant, K; Baird, K; Langford, CF; Gregory, SG; Collins, VP. 1p36 is a preferential target of chromosome 1 deletions in astrocytic tumours and homozygously deleted in a subset of glioblastomas. *Oncogene*, 2008, 27, 2097-2108.

[112] Idbaih, A; Kouwenhoven, M; Jeuken, J; Carpentier, C; Gorlia, T; Kros, JM; French, P; Teepen, JL; Delattre, O; Delattre, JY; van den Bent, M; Hoang-Xuan, K. Chromosome 1p loss evaluation in anaplastic oligodendrogliomas. *Neuropathology*, 2008, 28, 440-443.

[113] Jeuken, JW; Sprenger, SH; Wesseling, P; Macville, MV; von Deimling, A; Teepen, HL; van Overbeeke, JJ; Boerman, RH. Identification of subgroups of high-grade oligodendroglial tumors by comparative genomic hybridization. *Journal of Neuropathology and Experimental Neurology*, 1999, 58, 606-612.

[114] Jeuken, JW; Sprenger, SH; Boerman, RH; von Deimling, A; Teepen, HL; van Overbeeke, JJ; Wesseling, P. Subtyping of oligo-astrocytic tumours by comparative genomic hybridization. *The Journal of Pathology*, 2001, 194, 81-87.

[115] Jeuken, J; Cornelissen, S; Boots-Sprenger, S; Gijsen, S; Wesseling, P. Multiplex ligation-dependent probe amplification: a diagnostic tool for simultaneous identification of different genetic markers in glial tumors. *The Journal of Molecular Diagnostics*, 2006, 8, 433-443.

[116] Natté, R; van Eijk, R; Eilers, P; Cleton-Jansen, AM; Oosting, J; Kouwenhove, M; Kros, JM; van Duinen, S. Multiplex ligation-dependent probe amplification for the detection of 1p and 19q chromosomal loss in oligodendroglial tumors. *Brain Pathology*, 2005, 15, 192-197.

[117] Franco-Hernández, C; Martínez-Glez, V; de Campos, JM; Isla, A; Vaquero, J; Gutiérrez, M; Casartelli, C; Rey, JA. Allelic status of 1p and 19q in oligodendrogliomas and glioblastomas: multiplex ligation-dependent probe amplification versus loss of heterozygosity. *Cancer Genetics and Cytogenetics*, 2009, 190, 93-96.

[118] Dong, Z; Pang, JS; Ng, MH; Poon, WS; Zhou, L; Ng, HK. Identification of two contiguous minimally deleted regions on chromosome 1p36.31-p36.32 in oligodendroglial tumours. *British Journal of Cancer*, 2004, 91, 1105-1111.

[119] McDonald, JM; Dunmire, V; Taylor, E; Sawaya, R; Bruner, J; Fuller, GN; Aldape, K; Zhang, W. Attenuated expression of DFFB is a hallmark of oligodendrogliomas with 1p-allelic loss. *Molecular Cancer*, 2005, 4, 35.

[120] Tews, B; Felsberg, J; Hartmann, C; Kunitz, A; Hahn, M; Toedt, G; Neben, K; Hummerich, L; von Deimling, A; Reifenberger, G; Lichter, P. Identification of novel oligodendroglioma-associated candidate tumor suppressor genes in 1p36 and 19q13 using microarray-based expression profiling. *International Journal of Cancer*, 2006, 119, 792-800.

[121] Bello, MJ; de Campos, JM; Vaquero, J; Ruiz-Barnés, P; Kusak, ME; Sarasa, JL; Rey, JA. hRAD54 gene and 1p high-resolution deletion-mapping analyses in oligodendrogliomas. *Cancer Genetics and Cytogenetics*, 2000, 116, 142-147.

[122] Husemann, K; Wolter, M; Büschges, R; Boström, J; Sabel, M; Reifenberger, G. Identification of two distinct deleted regions on the short arm of chromosome 1 and rare mutation of the CDKN2C gene from 1p32 in oligodendroglial tumors. *Journal of Neuropathology and Experimental Neurology*, 1999, 58, 1041-1050.

[123] Pohl, U; Cairncross, JG; Louis, DN. Homozygous deletions of the CDKN2C/p18INK4C gene on the short arm of chromosome 1 in anaplastic oligodendrogliomas. *Brain Pathology*, 1999, 9, 639-643.

[124] Riemenschneider, MJ; Reifenberger, J; Reifenberger, G. Frequent biallelic inactivation and transcriptional silencing of the DIRAS3 gene at 1p31 in oligodendroglial tumors with 1p loss. *International Journal of Cancer*, 2008, 122, 2503-2510.

[125] Boulay, JL; Miserez, AR; Zweifel, C; Sivasankaran, B; Kana, V; Ghaffari, A; Luyken, C; Sabel, M; Zerrouqi, A; Wasner, M; Van Meir, E; Tolnay, M; Reifenberger, G; Merlo, A. Loss of NOTCH2 positively predicts survival in subgroups of human glial brain tumors. *PLoS One*, 2007, 2, e576.

[126] Zheng, S; Houseman, EA; Morrison, Z; Wrensch, MR; Patoka, JS; Ramos, C; Haas-Kogan, DA; McBride, S; Marsit, CJ; Christensen, BC; Nelson, HH; Stokoe,D; Wiemels, JL; Chang, SM; Prados, MD; Tihan, T; Vandenberg, SR; Kelsey, KT; Berger, MS; Wiencke, JK. DNA hypermethylation profiles associated with glioma subtypes and EZH2 and IGFBP2 mRNA expression. *Neuro Oncology*, 2011, 13, 280-289.

[127] Wolf, RM; Draghi, N; Liang, X; Dai, C; Uhrbom, L; Eklöf, C; Westermark, B; Holland, EC; Resh, MD. p190RhoGAP can act to inhibit PDGF-induced gliomas in mice: a putative tumor suppressor

encoded on human chromosome 19q13.3. *Genes & Development*, 2003, 17, 476-487.

[128] Kunitz, A; Wolter, M; van den Boom, J; Felsberg, J; Tews, B; Hahn, M; Benner, A; Sabel, M; Lichter, P; Reifenberger, G; von Deimling, A; Hartmann, C. DNA hypermethylation and aberrant expression of the EMP3 gene at 19q13.3 in Human Gliomas. *Brain Pathology*, 2007, 17, 363-370.

[129] Balss, J; Meyer, J; Mueller, W; Korshunov, A; Hartmann, C; von Deimling, A. Analysis of the IDH1 codon 132 mutation in brain tumors. *Acta Neuropathologica*, 2008, 116, 597-602.

[130] Mellai, M; Piazzi, A; Caldera, V; Monzeglio, O; Cassoni, P; Valente, G; Schiffer, D. IDH1 and IDH2 mutations, immunohistochemistry and associations in a series of brain tumors. *Journal of Neuro-Oncology*, 2011, 105, 345-357.

[131] Capper, D; Reuss, D; Schittenhelm, J; Hartmann, C; Bremer, J; Sahm, F; Harter, PN; Jeibmann, A; von Deimling, A. Mutation-specific IDH1 antibody differentiates oligodendrogliomas and oligoastrocytomas from other brain tumors with oligodendroglioma-like morphology. *Acta Neuropathologica*, 2011, 121, 241-252.

[132] Gravendeel, LA; Kloosterhof, NK; Bralten, LB; van Marion, R; Dubbink, HJ; Dinjens, W; Bleeker, FE; Hoogenraad, CC; Michiels, E; Kros, JM; van den Bent, M; Smitt, PA; French, PJ. Segregation of non-p.R132H mutations in IDH1 in distinct molecular subtypes of glioma. *Human Mutation*, 2010, 31, E1186-1199.

[133] Sun, H; Yin, L; Li, S; Han, S; Song, G; Liu, N; Yan, C. Prognostic significance of IDH mutation in adult low-grade gliomas: a meta-analysis. *Journal of Neuro-Oncology*, 2013, 113, 277-284.

[134] Wang, XW; Ciccarino, P; Rossetto, M; Boisselier, B; Marie, Y; Desestret, V; Gleize, V; Mokhtari, K; Sanson, M; Labussière, M. IDH mutations: genotype-phenotype correlation and prognostic impact. *BioMed Research International*, 2014, 2014, 540236.

[135] Lu, C; Ward, PS; Kapoor, GS; Rohle, D; Turcan, S; Abdel-Wahab, O; Edwards, CR; Khanin, R; Figueroa, ME; Melnick, A; Wellen, KE; O'Rourke, DM; Berger, SL; Chan, TA; Levine, RL; Mellinghoff, IK; Thompson, CB. IDH mutation impairs histone demethylation and results in a block to cell differentiation. *Nature*, 2012, 483, 474-478.

[136] Turcan, S; Rohle, D; Goenka, A; Walsh, LA; Fang, F; Yilmaz, E; Campos, C; Fabius, AW; Lu, C; Ward, PS; Thompson, CB; Kaufman, A; Guryanova, O; Levine, R; Heguy, A; Viale, A; Morris, LG; Huse, JT;

Mellinghoff, IK; Chan, TA. IDH1 mutation is sufficient to establish the glioma hypermethylator phenotype. *Nature*, 2012, 483, 479-483.

[137] Blackburn, EH. Structure and function of telomeres. *Nature*, 1991, 350, 569-573.

[138] Shay, JW; Bacchetti, S. A survey of telomerase activity in human cancer. *European Journal of Cancer*, 1997, 33, 787-791.

[139] Falchetti, ML; Larocca, LM; Pallini, R. Telomerase in brain tumors. *Child's Nervous System*, 2002, 18, 112-117.

[140] Labussière, M; Di Stefano, AL; Gleize, V; Boisselier, B; Giry, M; Mangesius, S; Bruno, A; Paterra, R; Marie, Y; Rahimian, A; Finocchiaro, G; Houlston, RS; Hoang-Xuan, K; Idbaih, A; Delattre, JY; Mokhtari, K; Sanson, M. TERT promoter mutations in gliomas, genetic associations and clinico-pathological correlations. *British Journal of Cancer,* 2014, 111, 2024-2032.

[141] Heidenreich, B; Rachakonda, PS; Hosen, I; Volz, F; Hemminki, K; Weyerbrock, A; Kumar, R. TERT promoter mutations and telomere length in adult malignant gliomas and recurrences. *Oncotarget*, 2015, 6, 10617-10633.

[142] Huang, DS; Wang, Z; He, XJ; Diplas, BH; Yang, R; Killela, PJ; Meng, Q; Ye, ZY; Wang, W; Jiang, XT; Xu, L; He, XL; Zhao, ZS; Xu, WJ; Wang, HJ; Ma, YY; Xia, YJ; Li, L; Zhang, RX; Jin, T; Zhao, ZK; Xu, J; Yu, S; Wu, F; Liang, J; Wang, S; Jiao, Y; Yan, H; Tao, HQ. Recurrent TERT promoter mutations identified in a large-scale study of multiple tumour types are associated with increased TERTexpression and telomerase activation. *European Journal of Cancer*, 2015, 51, 969-976.

[143] Killela, PJ; Reitman, ZJ; Jiao, Y; Bettegowda, C; Agrawal, N; Diaz, LA Jr; Friedman, AH; Friedman, H; Gallia, GL; Giovanella, BC; Grollman, AP; He, TC; He, Y; Hruban, RH; Jallo, GI; Mandahl, N; Meeker, AK; Mertens, F; Netto, GJ; Rasheed, BA; Riggins, GJ; Rosenquist, TA; Schiffman, M; Shih, IeM; Theodorescu, D; Torbenson, MS; Velculescu, VE; Wang, TL; Wentzensen, N; Wood, LD; Zhang, M; McLendon, RE; Bigner, DD; Kinzler, KW; Vogelstein, B; Papadopoulos, N; Yan, H. TERT promoter mutations occur frequently in gliomas and a subset of tumors derived from cells with low rates of self-renewal. *Proceedings of the National Academy of Sciences of the United States of America*, 2013, 110, 6021-6026.

[144] Koelsche, C; Sahm, F; Capper, D; Reuss, D; Sturm, D; Jones, DT; Kool, M; Northcott, PA; Wiestler, B; Böhmer, K; Meyer, J; Mawrin, C; Hartmann, C; Mittelbronn, M; Platten, M; Brokinkel, B; Seiz, M;

Herold-Mende, C; Unterberg, A; Schittenhelm, J; Weller, M; Pfister, S; Wick, W; Korshunov, A; von Deimling, A. Distribution of TERT promoter mutations in pediatric and adult tumors of the nervous system. *Acta Neuropathologica*, 2013, 126, 907-915.

[145] Chan, AK; Yao, Y; Zhang, Z; Chung, NY; Liu, JS; Li, KK; Shi, Z; Chan, DT; Poon, WS; Zhou, L; Ng, HK. TERT promoter mutations contribute to subset prognostication of lower-grade gliomas. *Modern Pathology*, 2015, 28, 177-186.

[146] Arita, H; Narita, Y; Fukushima, S; Tateishi, K; Matsushita, Y; Yoshida, A; Miyakita, Y; Ohno, M; Collins, VP; Kawahara, N; Shibui, S; Ichimura, K. Upregulating mutations in the TERT promoter commonly occur in adult malignant gliomas and are strongly associated with total 1p19q loss. *Acta Neuropathologica*, 2013, 126, 267-276.

[147] Goldberg, AD; Banaszynski, LA; Noh, KM; Lewis, PW; Elsaesser, SJ; Stadler, S; Dewel, S; Law, M; Guo, X, Li, X; Wen, D; Chapgier, A; DeKelver, RC; Miller, JC; Lee, YL; Boydston, EA; Holmes, MC; Gregory, PD; Greally, JM; Rafii, S; Yang, C; Scambler, PJ; Garrick, D; Gibbons, RJ; Higgs, DR; Cristea, IM; Urnov, FD; Zheng, D; Allis, CD. Distinct factors control histone variant H3.3 localization at specific genomic regions. *Cell*, 2010, 140, 678-691.

[148] Kannan, K; Inagaki, A; Silber, J; Gorovets, D; Zhang, J; Kastenhuber, ER; Heguy, A; Petrini, JH; Chan, TA; Huse, JT. Whole-exome sequencing identifies ATRX mutation as a key molecular determinant in lower-grade glioma. *Oncotarget*, 2012, 3, 1194-1203.

[149] Schwartzentruber, J; Korshunov, A; Liu, XY; Jones, DT; Pfaff, E; Jacob, K; Sturm, D; Fontebasso, AM; Quang, DA; Tönjes, M; Hovestadt, V; Albrecht, S; Kool, M; Nantel, A; Konermann, C; Lindroth, A; Jäger, N; Rausch, T; Ryzhova, M; Korbel, JO; Hielscher, T; Hauser, P; Garami, M; Klekner, A; Bognar, L; Ebinger, M; Schuhmann, MU; Scheurlen, W; Pekrun, A; Frühwald, MC; Roggendorf, W; Kramm, C; Dürken, M; Atkinson, J; Lepage, P; Montpetit, A; Zakrzewska, M; Zakrzewski, K; Liberski, PP; Dong, Z; Siegel, P; Kulozik, AE; Zapatka, M; Guha, A; Malkin, D; Felsberg, J; Reifenberger, G; von Deimling, A; Ichimura, K; Collins, VP; Witt, H; Milde, T; Witt, O; Zhang, C; Castelo-Branco, P; Lichter, P; Faury, D; Tabori, U; Plass, C; Majewski, J; Pfister, SM; Jabado, N. Driver mutations in histone H3.3 and chromatin remodelling genes in pediatric glioblastoma. *Nature*, 2012, 482, 226-231.

[150] Wiestler, B; Capper, D; Holland-Letz, T; Korshunov, A; von Deimling, A; Pfister, SM; Platten, M; Weller, M; Wick, W. ATRX loss refines the

classification of anaplastic gliomas and identifies a subgroup of IDH mutant astrocytic tumors with better prognosis. *Acta Neuropathologica*, 2013, 126, 443-451.

[151] Jiao, Y; Killela, PJ; Reitman, ZJ; Rasheed, AB; Heaphy, CM; de Wilde, RF; Rodriguez, FJ; Rosemberg, S; Oba-Shinjo, SM; Nagahashi Marie, SK; Bettegowda, C; Agrawal, N; Lipp, E; Pirozzi, C; Lopez, G; He, Y; Friedman, H; Friedman, AH; Riggins, GJ; Holdhoff, M; Burger, P; McLendon, R; Bigner, DD; Vogelstein, B; Meeker, AK; Kinzler, KW; Papadopoulos, N; Diaz, LA; Yan, H. Frequent ATRX, CIC, FUBP1 and IDH1 mutations refine the classification of malignant gliomas. *Oncotarget*, 2012, 3, 709-722.

[152] Liu, XY; Gerges, N; Korshunov, A; Sabha, N; Khuong-Quang, DA; Fontebasso, AM; Fleming, A; Hadjadj, D; Schwartzentruber, J; Majewski, J; Dong, Z; Siegel, P; Albrecht, S; Croul, S; Jones, DT; Kool, M; Tonjes, M; Reifenberger, G; Faury, D; Zadeh, G; Pfister, S; Jabado, N. Frequent ATRX mutations and loss of expression in adult diffuse astrocytic tumors carrying IDH1/IDH2 and TP53 mutations. *Acta Neuropathologica*, 2012, 124, 615-625.

[153] Cryan, JB; Haidar, S; Ramkissoon, LA; Bi, WL; Knoff, DS; Schultz, N; Abedalthagafi, M; Brown, L; Wen, PY; Reardon, DA; Dunn, IF; Folkerth, RD; Santagata, S; Lindeman, NI; Ligon, AH; Beroukhim, R; Hornick, JL; Alexander, BM; Ligon, KL; Ramkissoon, SH. Clinical multiplexed exome sequencing distinguishes adult oligodendroglial neoplasms from astrocytic and mixed lineage gliomas. *Oncotarget*, 2014, 5, 8083-8092.

[154] Wilcox, P; Li, CC; Lee, M; Shivalingam, B; Brennan, J; Suter, CM; Kaufman, K; Lum, T; Buckland, ME. Oligoastrocytomas: throwing the baby out with the bathwater? *Acta Neuropathologica*, 2015, 129, 147-149.

[155] Haberler, C; Wöhrer, A. Clinical Neuropathology practice news 2-2014: ATRX, a new candidate biomarker in gliomas. *Clinical Neuropathologica*, 2014, 33, 108-111.

[156] Leeper, HE; Caron, AA; Decker, PA; Jenkins, RB; Lachance, DH; Giannini, C. DH mutation, 1p19q codeletion and ATRX loss in WHO grade II gliomas. *Oncotarget*, 2015.

[157] Eisenreich, S; Abou-El-Ardat, K; Szafranski, K; Campos Valenzuela, JA; Rump, A; Nigro, JM; Bjerkvig, R; Gerlach, EM; Hackmann, K; Schröck, E; Krex D; Kaderali, L; Schackert, G; Platzer, M; Klink, B. Novel CIC point mutations and an exon-spanning, homozygous deletion

identified in oligodendroglial tumors by a comprehensive genomic approach including transcriptome sequencing. *PLoS One*, 2013, 8, e76623.

[158] Ajuria, L; Nieva, C; Winkler, C; Kuo, D; Samper, N; Andreu, MJ; Helman, A; González-Crespo, S; Paroush, Z; Courey, AJ; Jiménez, G. Capicua DNA-binding sites are general response elements for RTK signaling in Drosophila. *Development*, 2011, 138, 915-924.

[159] Dissanayake, K; Toth, R; Blakey, J; Olsson, O; Campbell, DG; Prescott, AR; MacKintosh, C. ERK/p90(RSK)/14-3-3 signalling has an impact on expression of PEA3 Ets transcription factors via the transcriptional repressor capicúa. *The Biochemical Journal*, 2011, 433, 515-525.

[160] Gleize, V; Alentorn, A; Connen de Kérillis, L; Labussière, M; Nadaradjane, AA; Mundwiller, E; Ottolenghi, C; Mangesius, S; Rahimian, A; Ducray, F; POLA network; Mokhtari, K; Villa, C; Sanson, M. CIC inactivating mutations identify aggressive subset of 1p19q codeleted gliomas. *Annals of Neurology*, 2015, 78, 355-374.

[161] Hsiao, HH; Nath, A; Lin, CY; Folta-Stogniew, EJ; Rhoades, E; Braddock, DT. Quantitative characterization of the interactions among c-myc transcriptional regulators FUSE, FBP, and FIR. *Biochemistry*, 2010, 49, 4620-4634.

[162] Dubbink, HJ; Atmodimedjo, PN; Kros, JM; French, PJ; Sanson, M; Idbaih, A; Wesseling, P; Enting, R; Spliet, W; Tijssen, C; Dinjens, WN; Gorlia, T; van den Bent, MJ. Molecular classification of anaplastic oligodendroglioma using next-generation sequencing: a report of the prospective randomized EORTC Brain Tumor Group 26951 phase III trial. *Neuro Oncology*, 2015.

[163] Hegi, ME; Diserens, AC; Gorlia, T; Hamou, MF; de Tribolet, N; Weller, M; Kros, JM; Hainfellner, JA; Mason, W; Mariani, L; Bromberg, JE; Hau, P; Mirimanoff, RO; Cairncross, JG; Janzer, RC; Stupp, R. MGMT gene silencing and benefit from temozolomide in glioblastoma. *The New England Journal of Medicine*, 2005, 352, 997-1003.

[164] Watanabe, T; Nakamura, M; Kros, JM; Burkhard, C; Yonekawa, Y; Kleihues, P; Ohgaki, H. Phenotype versus genotype correlation in oligodendrogliomas and low-grade diffuse astrocytomas. *Acta Neuropathologica,* 2002, 103, 267-275.

[165] Komine, C; Watanabe, T; Katayama, Y; Yoshino, A; Yokoyama, T; Fukushima, T. Promoter hypermethylation of the DNA repair gene O6-methylguanine-DNA methyltransferase is an independent predictor of

shortened progression-free survival in patients with low-grade diffuse astrocytomas. *Brain Pathology*, 2003, 13, 176-184.

[166] Möllemann, M; Wolter, M; Felsberg, J; Collins, VP; Reifenberger, G. Frequent promoter hypermethylation and low expression of the MGMT gene in oligodendroglial tumors. International journal of cancer. *Journal International du Cancer*, 2005, 113, 379-385.

[167] Mellai, M; Monzeglio, O; Piazzi, A; Caldera, V; Annovazzi, L; Cassoni, P; Valente, G; Cordera, S; Mocellini, C; Schiffer, D. MGMT promoter hypermethylation and its associations with genetic alterations in a series of 350 brain tumors. *Journal of Neurooncology*, 2012, 107, 617-631.

[168] Noushmehr, H; Weisenberger, DJ; Diefes, K; Phillips, HS; Pujara, K; Berman, BP; Pan, F; Pelloski, CE; Sulman, EP; Bhat, KP; Verhaak, RG; Hoadley, KA; Hayes, DN; Perou, CM; Schmidt, HK; Ding, L; Wilson, RK; Van Den Berg, D; Shen, H; Bengtsson, H; Neuvial, P; Cope, LM; Buckley, J; Herman, JG; Baylin, SB; Laird, PW; Aldape, K; Cancer Genome Atlas Research Network. Identification of a CpG island methylator phenotype that defines a distinct subgroup of glioma. *Cancer Cell,* 2010, 17, 510-522.

[169] van den Bent, MJ; Dubbink, HJ; Sanson, M; van der Lee-Haarloo, CR; Hegi, M; Jeuken, JW; Ibdaih, A; Brandes, AA; Taphoorn, MJ; Frenay, M; Lacombe, D; Gorlia, T; Dinjens, WN; Kros, JM. MGMT promoter methylation is prognostic but not predictive for outcome to adjuvant PCV chemotherapy in anaplastic oligodendroglial tumors: a report from EORTC Brain Tumor Group Study 26951. *Journal of Clinical Oncology*, 2009, 27, 5881-5886.

[170] Wick, W; Hartmann, C; Engel, C; Stoffels, M; Felsberg, J; Stockhammer, F; Sabe, MC; Koeppen, S; Ketter, R; Meyermann, R; Rapp, M; Meisner, C; Kortmann, RD; Pietsch, T; Wiestler, OD; Ernemann, U; Bamberg, M; Reifenberger, G; von Deimling, A; Weller, M. NOA-04 randomized phase III trial of sequential radiochemotherapy of anaplastic glioma with procarbazine, lomustine, and vincristine or temozolomide. *Journal of Clinical Oncology*, 2009, 27, 5874-5880.

[171] Wiestler, B; Capper, D; Hovestadt, V; Sill, M; Jones, DT; Hartmann, C; Felsberg, J; Platten, M; Feiden, W; Keyvani, K; Pfister, SM; Wiestler, OD; Meyermann, R; Reifenberger, G; Pietsch, T; von Deimling, A; Weller, M; Wick, W. Assessing CpG island methylator phenotype, 1p/19q codeletion, and MGMT promoter methylation from epigenome-wide data in the biomarker cohort of the NOA-04 trial. *Neuro Oncology*, 2014, 16, 1630-1638.

[172] Wick, W; Meisner, C; Hentschel, B; Platten, M; Schilling, A; Wiestler, B; Sabel, MC; Koeppen, S; Ketter, R; Weiler, M; Tabatabai, G; von Deimling, A; Gramatzki, D; Westphal, M; Schackert, G; Loeffler, M; Simon, M; Reifenberger, G; Weller, M. Prognostic or predictive value of MGMT promoter methylation in gliomas depends on IDH1 mutation. *Neurology*, 2013, 81, 1515-1522.

[173] van den Bent, MJ; Erdem-Eraslan, L; Idbaih, A; de Rooi, J; Eilers, PH; Spliet, WG; den Dunnen, WF; Tijssen, C; Wesseling, P; Sillevis Smitt, PA; Kros, JM; Gorlia, T; French, PJ. MGMT-STP27 methylation status as predictive marker for response to PCV in anaplastic Oligodendrogliomas and Oligoastrocytomas. A report from EORTC study 26951. *Clinical Cancer Research*, 2013, 19, 5513-5522.

[174] Preusser, M; Charles Janzer, R; Felsberg, J; Reifenberger, G; Hamou, MF; Diserens, AC; Stupp, R; Gorlia, T; Marosi, C; Heinzl, H; Hainfellner, JA; Hegi, M. Anti-O6-methylguanine-methyltransferase (MGMT) immunohistochemistry in glioblastoma multiforme: observer variability and lack of association with patient survival impede its use as clinical biomarker. *Brain Pathology*, 2008, 18, 520-532.

[175] Alaminos, M; Dávalos, V; Ropero, S; Setién, F; Paz, MF; Herranz, M; Fraga, MF; Mora, J; Cheung, NK; Gerald, WL; Esteller, M. EMP3, a myelin-related gene located in the critical 19q13.3 region, is epigenetically silenced and exhibits features of a candidate tumor suppressor in glioma and neuroblastoma. *Cancer Research,* 2005, 65, 2565-2571.

[176] Li, KK; Pang, JC; Chung, NY; Ng, YL; Chan, NH; Zhou, L; Poon, WS; Ng, HK. EMP3 overexpression is associated with oligodendroglial tumors retaining chromosome arms 1p and 19q. *International Journal of Cancer*, 2007, 120, 947-950.

[177] Taylor, V; Suter, U. Epithelial membrane protein-2 and epithelial membrane protein-3: two novel members of the peripheral myelin protein 22 gene family. *Gene*, 1996, 175, 115-120.

[178] Mellai, M; Piazzi, A; Caldera, V; Annovazzi, L; Monzeglio, O; Senetta, R; Cassoni, P; Schiffer, D. Promoter hypermethylation of the EMP3 gene in a series of 229 human gliomas. *BioMed Research International*, 2013, 2013, 756302.

[179] Fallon, KB; Palmer, CA; Roth, KA; Nabors, LB; Wang, W; Carpenter, M; Banerjee, R; Forsyth, P; Rich, K; Perry, A. Prognostic value of 1p, 19q, 9p, 10q, and EGFR-FISH analyses in recurrent oligodendrogliomas.

Journal of Neuropathology and Experimental Neurology, 2004, 63, 314-322.

[180] Broderick, DK; Di, C; Parrett, TJ; Samuels, YR; Cummins, JM; McLendon, RE; Fults, DW; Velculescu, VE; Bigner, DD; Yan, H. Mutations of PIK3CA in anaplastic oligodendrogliomas, high-grade astrocytomas, and medulloblastomas. *Cancer Research*, 2004, 64, 5048-5050.

[181] Agnihotri, S; Aldape, KD; Zadeh, G. Isocitrate dehydrogenase status and molecular subclasses of glioma and glioblastoma. *Neurosurgical Focus*, 2014, 37, E13.

[182] Cancer Genome Atlas Research Network. Comprehensive, Integrative Genomic Analysis of Diffuse Lower-Grade Gliomas. *The New England Journal of Medicine*, 2015, 372, 2481-2498.

[183] Snuderl, M; Eichler, AF; Ligon, KL; Vu, QU; Silver, M; Betensky, RA; Ligon, AH; Wen, PY; Louis, DN; Iafrate, AJ. Polysomy for chromosomes 1 and 19 predicts earlier recurrence in anaplastic oligodendrogliomas with concurrent 1p/19q loss. *Clinical Cancer Research*, 2009, 15, 6430-6437.

[184] Ren, X; Jiang, H; Cui, X; Cui, Y; Ma, J; Jiang, Z; Sui, D; Lin, S. Co-polysomy of chromosome 1q and 19p predicts worse prognosis in 1p/19q codeleted oligodendroglial tumors: FISH analysis of 148 consecutive cases. *Neuro Oncology*, 2013, 15, 1244-1250.

[185] Labreche, K; Simeonova, I; Kamoun, A; Gleize, V; Chubb, D; Letouzé, E; Riazalhosseini, Y; Dobbins, SE; Elarouci, N; Ducray, F; de Reyniès, A; Zelenika, D; Wardell, CP; Frampton, M; Saulnier, O; Pastinen, T; Hallout, S; Figarella-Branger, D; Dehais, C; Idbaih, A; Mokhtari, K; Delattre, JY; Huillard, E; Mark Lathrop, G; Sanson, M; Houlston, RS; POLA Network. TCF12 is mutated in anaplastic oligodendroglioma. *Nature Communications,* 2015, 6, 7207.

[186] Uittenbogaard, M; Chiaramello, A. Expression of the bHLH transcription factor Tcf12 (ME1) gene is linked to the expansion of precursor cell populations during neurogenesis. *Brain Research. Gene Expression Patterns*, 2002, 1, 115-121.

[187] Fu, H; Cai, J; Clevers, H; Fast, E; Gray, S; Greenberg, R; Jain, MK; Ma, Q; Qiu, M; Rowitch, DH; Taylor, CM; Stiles, CD. A genome-wide screen for spatially restricted expression patterns identifies transcription factors that regulate glial development. *The Journal of Neuroscience*, 2009, 29, 11399-11408.

[188] Kreiger, PA; Okada, Y; Simon, S; Rorke, LB; Louis, DN; Golden, JA. Losses of chromosomes 1p and 19q are rare in pediatric oligodendrogliomas. *Acta Neuropathologica,* 109, 387-392.

[189] Rodriguez, FJ; Tihan, T; Lin, D; McDonald, W; Nigro, J; Feuerstein, B; Jackson, S; Cohen, K; Burger, PC. Clinicopathologic features of pediatric oligodendrogliomas: a series of 50 patients. *The American Journal of Surgical Pathology*, 2014, 38, 1058-1070.

[190] Suri, V; Jha, P; Agarwal, S; Pathak, P; Sharma, MC; Sharma, V; Shukla, S; Somasundaram, K; Mahapatra, AK; Kale, SS; Sarkar, C. Molecular profile of oligodendrogliomas in young patients. *Neuro Oncology*, 2011, 13, 1099-1106.

[191] Sturm, D; Witt, H; Hovestadt, V; Khuong-Quang, DA; Jones, DT; Konermann, C; Pfaff, E; Tönjes, M; Sill, M; Bender, S; Kool, M; Zapatka, M; Becker, N; Zucknick, M; Hielscher, T; Liu, XY; Fontebasso, AM; Ryzhova, M; Albrecht, S; Jacob, K; Wolter, M; Ebinger, M; Schuhmann, MU; van Meter, T; Frühwald, MC; Hauch, H; Pekrun, A; Radlwimmer, B; Niehues, T; von Komorowski, G; Dürken, M; Kulozik, AE; Madden, J; Donson, A; Foreman, NK; Drissi, R; Fouladi, M; Scheurlen, W; von Deimling, A; Monoranu, C; Roggendorf, W; Herold-Mende, C; Unterberg, A; Kramm, CM; Felsberg, J; Hartmann, C; Wiestler, B; Wick, W; Milde, T; Witt, O; Lindroth, AM; Schwartzentruber, J; Faury, D; Fleming, A; Zakrzewska, M; Liberski, PP; Zakrzewski, K; Hauser, P; Garami, M; Klekner, A; Bognar, L; Morrissy, S; Cavalli, F; Taylor, MD; van Sluis, P; Koster, J; Versteeg, R; Volckmann, R; Mikkelsen, T; Aldape, K; Reifenberger, G; Collins, VP; Majewski, J; Korshunov, A; Lichter, P; Plass, C; Jabado, N; Pfister, SM. Hotspot mutations in H3F3A and IDH1 define distinct epigenetic and biological subgroups of glioblastoma. *Cancer Cell*, 2012, 22, 425-437.

[192] Gajjar, A; Pfister, SM; Taylor, MD; Gilbertson, RJ. Molecular insights into pediatric brain tumors have the potential to transform therapy. *Clinical Cancer Research*, 2014, 20, 5630-5640.

[193] Kim, YH; Nonoguchi, N; Paulus, W; Brokinkel, B; Keyvani, K; Sure, U; Wrede, K; Mariani, L; Giangaspero, F; Tanaka, Y; Nakazato, Y; Vital, A; Mittelbronn, M; Perry, A; Ohgaki, H. Frequent BRAF gain in low-grade diffuse gliomas with 1p/19q loss. *Brain Pathology*, 2012, 22, 834-840.

[194] Badiali, M; Gleize, V; Paris, S; Moi, L; Elhouadani, S; Arcella, A; Morace R; Antonelli, M; Buttarelli, FR; Figarella-Branger, D; Kim, YH;

Ohgaki, H; Mokhtari, K; Sanson, M; Giangaspero, F. KIAA1549-BRAF fusions and IDH mutations can coexist in diffuse gliomas of adults. *Brain Pathology*, 2012, 22, 841-847.

[195] Kumar, A; Pathak, P; Purkait, S; Faruq, M; Jha, P; Mallick, S; Suri, V; Sharma, MC; Suri, A; Sarkar, C. Oncogenic KIAA1549-BRAF fusion with activation of the MAPK/ERK pathway in pediatric oligodendrogliomas. *Cancer Genetics*, 2015, 208, 91-95.

[196] Rodriguez, FJ; Schniederjan, MJ; Nicolaides, T; Tihan, T; Burger, PC; Perry, A; High rate of concurrent BRAF-KIAA1549 gene fusion and 1p deletion in disseminated oligodendroglioma-like leptomeningeal neoplasms (DOLN). *Acta Neuropathologica*, 2015, 129, 609-610.

[197] Myung, JK; Cho, HJ; Kim, H; Park, CK; Lee, SH; Choi, SH; Park, P; Yoon, JM; Park, SH. Prognosis of Glioblastoma With Oligodendroglioma Component is Associated With the IDH1 Mutation and MGMT Methylation Status. *Translational Oncology*, 2014, 7 712-719.

[198] Kraus, JA; Lamszus, K; Glesmann, N; Beck, M; Wolter, M; Sabel, M; Krex, D; Klockgether, T; Reifenberger, G; Schlegel, U. Molecular genetic alterations in glioblastomas with oligodendroglial component. *Acta Neuropathologica,* 2001 101, 311-320.

[199] He, J; Mokhtari, K; Sanson, M; Marie, Y; Kujas, M; Huguet, S; Leuraud, P; Capelle, L; Delattre, JY; Poirier, J; Hoang-Xuan, K. Glioblastomas with an oligodendroglial component: a pathological and molecular study. *Journal of Neuropathology and Experimental Neurology*, 2001, 60, 863-871.

[200] Laxton, RC; Popov, S; Doey, L; Jury, A; Bhangoo, R; Gullan, R; Chandler, C; Brazil, L; Sadler, G; Beaney, R; Sibtain, N; King, A; Bodi, I; Jones, C; Ashkan, K; Al-Sarraj, S. Primary glioblastoma with oligodendroglial differentiation has better clinical outcome but no difference in common biological markers compared with other types of glioblastoma. *Neuro Oncology*, 2013, 15, 1635-1643.

[201] Joseph, NM; Phillips, J; Dahiya, SM; Felicella, M; Tihan, T; Brat, DJ; Perry, A. Diagnostic implications of IDH1-R132H and OLIG2 expression patterns in rare and challenging glioblastoma variants. *Modern Pathology*, 2013, 26, 315-326.

[202] Mizoguchi, M; Hata, N; Suzuki, SO; Fujioka, Y; Murata, H; Amano, T; Nakamizo, A; Yoshimoto, K; Iwaki, T; Sasaki, T. Pediatric glioblastoma with oligodendroglioma component: aggressive clinical phenotype with distinct molecular characteristics. *Neuropathology*, 2013, 33, 652-657.

[203] Homma, T; Fukushima, T; Vaccarella, S; Yonekawa, Y; Di Patre, PL; Franceschi, S; Ohgaki, H. Correlation among pathology, genotype, and patient outcomes in glioblastoma. *Journal of Neuropathology and Experimental Neurology*, 2006, 65, 846-854.

[204] Watanabe, T; Nobusawa, S; Kleihues, P; Ohgaki, H. IDH1 mutations are early events in the development of astrocytomas and oligodendrogliomas. *The American Journal of Pathology*, 2009, 174, 1149-1153.

[205] Wang, XW; Ciccarino, P; Rossetto, M; Boisselier, B; Marie, Y; Desestret, V; Gleize, V; Mokhtari, K; Sanson, M; Labussière, M. IDH mutations: genotype-phenotype correlation and prognostic impact. *BioMed Research International*, 2014, 2014, 540236.

[206] Appin, CL; Brat, DJ. Molecular pathways in gliomagenesis and their relevance to neuropathologic diagnosis. *Advances in Anatomic Pathology*, 2015, 22, 50-58.

[207] Groenendijk, FH; Taal, W; Dubbink, HJ; Haarloo, CR; Kouwenhoven, MC; van den Bent, MJ; Kros, JM; Dinjens, WN. MGMT promoter hypermethylation is a frequent, early, and consistent event in astrocytoma progression, and not correlated with TP53 mutation. *Journal of Neurooncology*, 2011, 101, 405-417.

[208] Kozomara, A; Griffiths-Jones, S. miRBase: integrating microRNA annotation and deep-sequencing data. *Nucleic Acids Research*, 2011, 39 (Database issue), D152-157.

[209] Lages, E; Guttin, A; El Atifi, M; Ramus, C; Ipas, H; Dupré, I; Rolland, D; Salon, C; Godfraind, C; deFraipont, F; Dhobb, M; Pelletier, L; Wion, D; Gay, E; Berger, F; Issartel, JP. MicroRNA and target protein patterns reveal physiopathological features of glioma subtypes. *PLoS One*, 2011, 6, e20600.

[210] Nelson, PT; Baldwin, DA; Kloosterman, WP; Kauppinen, S; Plasterk, RH; Mourelatos, Z. RAKE and LNA-ISH reveal microRNA expression and localization in archival human brain. *RNA*, 2006, 12, 187-191.

[211] Kim, G; Park, EC; Ryu CH; Jeon, SS; Kim, II; Jang, HS; Kim, GH; Choi, BO. MicroRNA expression profiling in recurrent anaplastic oligodendroglioma treated with postoperative radiotherapy, *Journal of Analytical Science & Technology*, 2011, 2, 97-104.

[212] Li, KK; Yang, L; Pang, JC; Chan, AK; Zhou, L; Mao, Y; Wang, Y; Lau, KM; Poon, WS; Shi, Z; Ng, HK. MIR-137 Suppresses Growth and Invasion, is Downregulated in Oligodendroglial Tumors and Targets CSE1L. *Brain Pathology*, 2013, 23, 426-439.

[213] Dehghani, F; Schachenmayr, W; Laun, A; Korf, HW. Prognostic implication of histopathological, immunohistochemical and clinical features of oligodendrogliomas: a study of 89 cases. *Acta Neuropathologica*, 1998, 95, 493-504.

[214] Olson, JD; Riedel, E; DeAngelis, LM. Long-term outcome of low-grade oligodendroglioma and mixed glioma. *Neurology*, 2000, 54, 1442-1448.

[215] Wharton, SB; Hamilton, FA; Chan, WK; Chan, KK; Anderson, JR. Proliferation and cell death in oligodendrogliomas. *Neuropathology and Applied Neurobiology*, 1998 24, 21-28.

[216] Yeh, SA; Lee, TC; Chen, HJ; Lui, CC; Sun, LM; Wang, CJ; Huang, EY. Treatment outcomes and prognostic factors of patients with supratentorial low-grade oligodendroglioma. *International Journal of Radiation Oncology, Biology, Physics*, 2002, 54, 1405-1409.

[217] Puduvalli, VK; Hashmi, M; McAllister, LD; Levin, VA; Hess, KR; Prados, M; Jaeckle, KA; Yung, WK; Buys, SS; Bruner, JM; Townsend, JJ; Davis, R; Sawaya, R; Kyritsis, AP. Anaplastic oligodendrogliomas: prognostic factors for tumor recurrence and survival. *Oncology*, 2003, 65, 259-266.

[218] Shaw, EG; Wang, M; Coons, SW; Brachman, DG; Buckner, JC; Stelzer, KJ; Barger, GR; Brown, PD; Gilbert, MR; Mehta, MP. Randomized trial of radiationtherapy plus procarbazine, lomustine, and vincristine chemotherapy for supratentorial adult low-grade glioma: initial results of RTOG 9802. *Journal of Clinical Oncology*, 2012, 30, 3065-3070.

[219] Jeremic, B; Jovanovic, D; Djuric, LJ; Jevremovic, S; Mijatovic, LJ. Advantage of post-radiotherapy chemotherapy with CCNU, procarbazine, and vincristine (mPCV) over chemotherapy with VM-26 and CCNU for malignant gliomas. *Journal of Chemotherapy*, 1992, 4, 123-126.

[220] Kappelle, AC; Postma, TJ; Taphoorn, MJ; Groeneveld, GJ; van den Bent MJ; van Groeningen, CJ; Zonnenberg, BA; Sneeuw, KC; Heimans, JJ. PCV chemotherapy for recurrent glioblastoma multiforme. *Neurology*, 2001, 56, 118-120.

[221] Levin, VA; Uhm, JH; Jaeckle, KA; Choucair, A; Flynn, PJ; Yung, WKA; Prados, MD; Bruner, JM; Chang, SM, Kyritsis, AP; Gleason, MJ; Hess, KR. Phase III randomized study of postradiotherapy chemotherapy with alpha-difluoromethylornithine-procarbazine, N-(2-chloroethyl)-N'-cyclohexyl-N-nitrosurea, vincristine (DFMO-PCV) versus PCV for glioblastoma multiforme. *Clinical Cancer Research*, 2000, 6, 3878-3884.

[222] Levin, VA; Hess, KR; Choucair, A; Flynn, PJ; Jaeckle, KA; Kyritsis, AP; Yung, WK; Prados, MD; Bruner, JM; Ictech, S; Gleason, MJ; Kim, HW. Phase III randomized study of postradiotherapy chemotherapy with combination alpha-difluoromethylornithine-PCV versus PCV for anaplastic gliomas. *Clinical Cancer Research*, 2003, 9, 981-990.
[223] van den Bent, MJ; Brandes, AA; Taphoorn, MJ; Kros, JM; Kouwenhoven, MC; Delattre, JY; Bernsen, HJ; Frenay, M; Tijssen, CC; Grisold, W; Sipos, L; Enting, RH; French, PJ; Dinjens, WN; Vecht, CJ; Allgeier, A; Lacombe, D; Gorlia, T; Hoang-Xuan, K. Adjuvant procarbazine, lomustine, and vincristine chemotherapy in newly diagnosed anaplastic oligodendroglioma: long-term follow-up of EORTC brain tumor group study 26951. *Journal of Clinical Oncology*, 2013, 31, 344-350.
[224] Lebrun, C; Fontaine, D; Bourg, V; Ramaioli, A; Chanalet, S; Vandenbos, F; Lonjon, M; Fauchon, F; Paquis, P; Frenay, M. Treatment of newly diagnosed symptomatic pure low-grade oligodendrogliomas with PCV chemotherapy. *European Journal of Neurology*. 2007, 14, 391-398.
[225] Buckner, JC; Pugh, SL; Shaw, EG; Gilbert, MR; Barger, G; Coons, S; Ricci, P; Bullard, D; Brown, PD; Stelzer, K; Brachman, D; Suh, JH; Schultz, CJ; Bahary, JP; Fisher, BJ; Kim, H; Murtha, AD; Curran, WJ; Mehta, MP. Phase III study of radiation therapy (RT) with or without procarbazine, CCNU, and vincristine (PCV) in low-grade glioma: RTOG 9802 with Alliance, ECOG, and SWOG. *Journal of Clinical Oncology*, 2014, 32, 5s.
[226] Cairncross, G; Berkey, B; Shaw, E; Jenkins, R; Scheithauer, B; Brachman, D; Buckner, J; Fink, K; Souhami, L; Laperierre, N; Mehta, M; Curran, W. Phase III trial of chemotherapy plus radiotherapy compared with radiotherapy alone for pure and mixed anaplastic oligodendroglioma: Intergroup Radiation Therapy Oncology Group Trial 9402. *Journal of Clinical Oncology*, 2006, 24, 2707-2714.
[227] Cairncross, G; Macdonald, D; Ludwin, S; Lee, D; Cascino, T; Buckner, J; Fulton, D; Dropcho, E; Stewart, D; Schold, C; Jr. et al. Chemotherapy for anaplastic oligodendroglioma. National Cancer Institute of Canada Clinical Trials Group. *Journal of Clinical Oncology*, 1994, 12, 2013-2021.
[228] Shaw, EG; Scheithauer, BW; O'Fallon, JR; Tazelaar, HD; Davis, DH. Oligodendrogliomas: the Mayo Clinic experience. *Journal of Neurosurgery*, 1992, 76, 428-434.

[229] Winger, MJ; Macdonald, DR; Cairncross, JG. Supratentorial anaplastic gliomas in adults. The prognostic importance of extent of resection and prior low-grade glioma. *Journal of Neurosurgery*, 1989, 71, 487-493.

[230] Jiang, H; Ren, X; Wang, J; Zhang, Z; Jia, W; Lin, S. Short-term survivors in glioblastomas with oligodendroglioma component: a clinical study of 186 Chinese patients from a single institution. *Journal of Neurooncology*, 2014, 116, 395-404.

[231] Levin, N; Lavon, I; Zelikovitsh, B; Fuchs, D; Bokstein, F; Fellig, Y; Siegal, T. Progressive low-grade oligodendrogliomas: response to temozolomide and correlation between genetic profile and O6-methylguanine DNA methyltransferase protein expression. *Cancer*, 2006, 106, 1759-1765.

[232] Brandner, S; von Deimling, A. Diagnostic, prognostic and predictive relevance of molecular markers in gliomas. *Neuropathology and Applied Neurobiology*, 2015, 41, 694-720.

[233] Wick, W; Hartmann, C; Engel, C; Stoffels, M; Felsberg, J; Stockhammer, F; Sabel, MC; Koeppen, S; Ketter, R; Meyermann, R; Rapp, M; Meisner, C; Kortmann, RD; Pietsch, T; Wiestler, OD; Ernemann, U; Bamberg, M; Reifenberger, G; von Deimling, A; Weller, M. NOA-04 randomized phase III trial of sequential radiochemotherapy of anaplastic glioma with procarbazine, lomustine, and vincristine or temozolomide. *Journal of Clinical Oncology*, 2009, 27, 5874-5880.

[234] van den Bent, MJ; Brandes, AA; Taphoorn, MJ; Kros, JM; Kouwenhoven, MC; Delattre, JY; Bernsen, HJ; Frenay, M; Tijssen, CC; Grisold, W; Sipos, L; Enting, RH; French, PJ; Dinjens, WN; Vecht, CJ; Allgeier, A; Lacombe, D; Gorlia, T; Hoang-Xuan, K. Adjuvant procarbazine, lomustine, and vincristine chemotherapy in newly diagnosed anaplastic oligodendroglioma: long-term follow-up of EORTC brain tumor group study 26951. *Journal of Clinical Oncology,* 2013, 31, 344-350.

[235] Cairncross, G; Wang, M; Shaw, E; Jenkins, R; Brachman, D; Buckner, J; Fink, K; Souhami, L; Laperriere, N; Curran, W; Mehta, M. Phase III trial of chemoradiotherapy for anaplastic oligodendroglioma: long-term results of RTOG 9402. *Journal of Clinical Oncology*, 2013, 31, 337-343.

[236] Brandes, AA; Tosoni, A; Cavallo, G; Reni, M; Franceschi, E; Bonaldi, L; Bertorelle, R; Gardiman, M; Ghimenton, C; Iuzzolino, P; Pession, A; Blatt, V; Ermani, M; GICNO. Correlations between O6-methylguanine DNA methyltransferase promoter methylation status, 1p and 19q deletions, and response to temozolomide in anaplastic and recurrent

oligodendroglioma: a prospective GICNO study. *Journal of Clinical Oncology*, 2006, 24, 4746-4753.

[237] Kouwenhoven, MC; Kros, JM; French, PJ; Biemond-ter Stege, EM; Graveland, WJ; Taphoorn, MJ; Brandes, AA; van den Bent, MJ. 1p/19q loss within oligodendroglioma is predictive for response to first line temozolomide but not to salvage treatment. *European Journal of Cancer*, 2006, 42, 2499-2503.

[238] Speirs, CK; Simpson, JR; Robinson, CG; DeWees, TA; Tran, DD; Linette, G; Chicoine, MR; Dacey, RG; Rich, KM; Dowling, JL; Leuthardt, EC; Zipfel, GJ; Kim, AH; Huang, J. Impact of 1p/19q codeletion and histology *International Iournal of Radiation Oncology, Biology, Physics*, 2015, 91, 268-276.

[239] Houillier, C; Wang, X; Kaloshi, G; Mokhtari, K; Guillevin, R; Laffaire, J; Paris, S; Boisselier, B; Idbaih, A; Laigle-Donadey, F; Hoang-Xuan, K; Sanson, M; Delattre, JY. IDH1 or IDH2 mutations predict longer survival and response to temozolomide in low-grade gliomas. *Neurology*, 2010, 75, 1560-1566.

[240] Cairncross, JG; Wang, M; Jenkins, RB; Shaw, EG; Giannini, C; Brachman, DG; Buckner, JC; Fink, KL; Souhami, L; Laperriere, NJ; Huse, JT; Mehta, MP; Curran, WJ Jr. Benefit from procarbazine, lomustine, and vincristine in oligodendroglial tumors is associated with mutation of IDH. *Journal of Clinical Oncology*, 2014, 32, 783-790.

[241] van den Bent, MJ; Gravendeel, LA; Gorlia, T; Kros, JM; Lapre, L; Wesseling, P; Teepen, JL; Idbaih, A; Sanson, M; Smitt, PA; French, PJ. A hypermethylated phenotype is a better predictor of survival than MGMT methylation in anaplastic oligodendroglial brain tumors: a report from EORTC study 26951. *Clinical Cancer Research*, 2011, 17, 7148-7155.

[242] Hoang-Xuan, K; He, J; Huguet, S; Mokhtari, K; Marie, Y; Kujas, M; Leuraud, P; Capelle, L; Delattre, JY; Poirier, J; Broët, P; Sanson, M. Molecular heterogeneity of oligodendrogliomas suggests alternative pathways in tumor progression. *Neurology*, 2001, 57, 1278-1281.

[243] Idbaih, A; Dalmasso, C; Kouwenhoven, M; Jeuken, J; Carpentier, C; Gorlia, T; Kros, JM; French, P; Teepen, J; Broët, P; Delattre, O; Mokhtari, K; Sanson, M; Delattre, JY; van den Bent, M; Hoang-Xuan, K. Genomic aberrations associated with outcome in anaplastic oligodendroglial tumors treated within the EORTC phase III trial 26951. *Journal of NeurooOncology*, 2011 103, 221-230.

[244] Cairncross, JG; Macdonald, DR. Successful chemotherapy for recurrent malignant oligodendroglioma. *Annals of Neurology*, 1988, 23 360-364.

[245] Bortolotto, S; Chiadò-Piat, L; Cavalla, P; Bosone, I; Chiò, A; Mauro, A; Schiffer, D. CDKN2A/p16 inactivation in the prognosis of oligodendrogliomas. *International Journal of Cancer*, 2000, 88, 554-557.

[246] McLendon, RE; Herndon, JE 2nd; West, B; Reardon, D; Wiltshire, R; Rasheed, BK; Quinn, J; Friedman, HS; Friedman, AH; Bigner, DD. Survival analysis of presumptive prognostic markers among oligodendrogliomas. *Cancer*, 2005, 104, 1693-1699.

[247] Ramirez, C; Bowman, C; Maurage, CA; Dubois, F; Blond, S; Porchet, N; Escande, F. Loss of 1p, 19q, and 10q heterozygosity prospectively predicts prognosis of oligodendroglial tumors--towards individualized tumor treatment? *Neuro Oncology*, 2010, 12, 490-499.

In: Oligodendrogliomas (ODs)
Editor: Chad Reeves

ISBN: 978-1-63484-278-5

Chapter 2

MOLECULAR MARKERS OF OLIGODENDROGLIOMAS

Tomaz Velnar
Department of Neurosurgery,
University Medical Centre Ljubljana, Ljubljana, Slovenia

ABSTRACT

Oliogodendroglial tumours arise from oligodendroglial cells or their precursors. Typically located in cerebral hemispheres, they are diffusely infiltrating neoplasms, either well differentiated or with focal or diffuse features of malignancy. Oligodendrogliomas represent the third most common glial tumour and account for 5% of primary brain neoplasms. Besides predicting the tumour sensitivity to chemotherapy, the 1p and 19q mutations that are most frequently found in oligodendrogliomas may be useful to determine the type of tumour in morphologically ambiguous cases, as no immunohistological markers for oligodendrogliomas are known so far. In this chapter, the oligodendrogliomas and the problematic of diagnostic markers are shortly discussed.

INTRODUCTION

Cancer is the second leading cause of morbidity and mortality worldwide, ranking just after cardiovascular diseases [1]. In the central nervous system, gliomas constitute the most frequent type of tumours. According to the cell origin, they may be divided into astrocytomas, oligodendroglial tumours and mixed gliomas [2, 3].

The prognosis of cancer patients has improved as a result of remarkable progress in the aspects of cancer treatment that was made over the past decade. Especially important are the advances in imaging methods, surgical and chemotherapeutic techniques, radiation delivery, as well as in the patohistological diagnosis and development in molecular biology [3-5]. However, despite optimal diagnostics and treatment, cancer burden in the society is still ranking too high [2, 6].

According to the definition, oligodendrogliomas are diffusely infiltrating glial tumours, composed of neoplastic oligodendroglial cells, typically found in cerebral hemispheres in adult population, although not uncommon in children. They encompass a range of tumours, from well-differentiated to frankly malignant neoplasms. In the current World Health Organization (WHO) classification of tumours of the central nervous system, covering a four-tiered WHO grading scheme, oligodendrogliomas are recognised as grade WHO II and WHO III by the degree of malignancy. They may be either well differentiated, composed of neoplastic cells that morphologically resemble oligodendroglia, or may harbour focal or diffuse features of malignancy, respectively. Their prognosis is in this case less favourable [7].

As histologically identical tumours may exhibit different treatment outcomes, the molecular markers carry both diagnostic and prognostic information and are a valuable tool for both tumour identification and assessment in modern neurooncology. In the past twenty years, oligodendrogliomas have gained much interest due to a favourable treatment response to chemotherapy. The biomarker status now helps to guide the clinical decisions in oligodendrogliomas. According to the molecular and biological characteristics, oligodendrogliomas may be additionally subdivided into prognostic subgroups with the benefit in terms of overall survival and progression-free survival [8-11]. Together with clinical and histological factors, they may all define the appropriate antitumor therapy and predict the outcome of treatment [7, 8, 12, 13].

EPIDEMIOLOGY AND AETIOLOGY

Oliogodendrogliomas arise from oligodendroglial cells or their precursors and represent the third most frequent type of glial tumours, ranking closely after glioblastoma multiforme and astrocytomas. They constitute 5% to 20% of gliomas and 5% to 25% of primary tumours found in the brain [2, 6, 8, 14-16]. The annual incidence rate of oligodendrogliomas is two to four per 1000000 people. The incidence is increasing every year [2, 6]. It is believed that one of the main reasons these tumours are encountered more common than once thought, are the improved diagnostic methods, including preoperative imaging and histological and molecular techniques. Many tumours in the past were diagnosed as astrocytomas of various types, although in reality they were oligodendrogliomas. Thus, improved techniques, especially magnetic resonance imaging and better histological recognition have contributed to a rise in the incidence [2, 6, 16-18].

Although oligodendrogliomas may occur at any age, they are most frequently found in the adult population. However, there are two periods of age when the tumours are diagnosed more frequently and these periods differ according to literature reports. The first peak of incidence is reported between six and 12 years, where oligodendrogliomas represent 1% of childhood brain tumours. The second peak is between 35 and 45 years [2]. Both genders may be affected with the male-to-female ratio of 1.5 to 1. In males, peak incidence was described between 45 to 49 years and in females between 55 to 59 years [2, 6]. In younger patients, low grade oligodendrogliomas predominate. Also familial clustering of tumours was found, with no genetic factors nor special pattern of inheritance until now [19-21]. Furthermore, causes for oligodendroglioma evolvement are unknown. There were no lifestyle or environmental factors discovered so far [6, 19, 22, 23].

The tumour may evolve at any location where oligodendrocytes are found. More than 90% of oligodendrogliomas arise supratentorially in the cortex and cerebral white matter, rarely in deep cerebral structures. The frontal lobe is affected in 60% of cases. In decreasing frequencies, the temporal, parietal and occipital lobes follow in 47%, 20% and 4%, respectively. Involvement of more than one cerebral lobe or multifocal localisation is rare. In the infratentorial sites and in the brainstem and spinal cord, less than 10% of oligodendrogliomas have been reported [2, 6, 21].

TUMOUR SIGNS AND SYMPTOMS

The symptoms of oligodendroglial tumours are comparable to other primary brain neoplasms. The most common symptom are the epileptic seizures, presenting in 35% to 85% of patients. Seizures may be generalised, simple or complex partial, or a combination of these [2, 18, 24]. They may be experienced for a number of years before the diagnosis, although with the use of computed tomography and magnetic resonance imaging the intervals this situation is less common [24-27]. Other symptoms include headaches, sensory and motor disturbances in terms of localised limb weakness, visual complaints, nausea, dizziness and sudden or insidious change in personality and mood. It is not uncommon that symptoms precede the definitive diagnosis with their average duration of 3 months to 5 years [2, 16, 26, 27].

Oligodendrogliomas may sometimes invade meninges [2]. Besides medulloblastomas, there is also in oligodendrogliomas a tendency to disseminate through cerebrospinal fluid and to develop drop metastasis or leptomeningeal seeding along the neuraxis [28]. This is a delayed complication described in 1% to 2% of patients [6, 28]. Very rarely, the tumours may spread to other locations, receiving the highest blood flow in the body, such as lung, liver and bone [29]. Due to improved survival of oligodendroglioma patients, metastatic disease is encountered more frequently [2, 6].

Treatment of Oligodendroglial Tumours

There are three therapeutic modalities for treatment of oligodendrogliomas that are connected and combinable. They include surgery, radiation therapy and chemotherapy [2, 6]. All three are often used successively. Surgery remains most frequently employed method both in order to perform a tumour reduction or a gross resection where possible and to obtain tissue samples for the definite diagnosis [6, 24, 30, 31]. The resection decreases the tumour mass effect on the brain with concomitant neurological consequences and reduces the tumour load during radiotherapy, which is the next and often following form of treatment [32, 33]. Radiotherapy is used due to an invasive nature of tumour growth where deep infiltration of tumour cells cannot be determined during surgery and therefore a complete removal is not possible. As a consequence, the disease relapses slowly but inevitably [33, 34]. A tumour recurrence takes place at the operative site. It may have the form of a high grade tumour, an anaplastic oligodendroglioma or even glioblastoma. While low-grade tumours may recur after many years, anaplastic ones tend to do so sooner. Additionally, metastases through the cerebrospinal fluid have also been described [2, 24, 16]. The third option of treatment is chemotherapy, which is being widely used. On the contrary to low-grade oligodendrogliomas, where radiation is delayed until tumour progression, patents with anaplastic oligodendrogliomas receive both radiation and chemotherapy and this combination is superior to either treatment alone [2, 6, 32, 33]. A reason of increasingly employed chemotherapy comes from the observations that low-grade and anaplastic oligodendrogliomas are chemosensitive tumours. Chemotherapy is used as a treatment option and with or without radiotherapy, the latter option in children, where radiation is usually withheld due to adverse effects on the developing nervous system. Chemotherapy application before radiotherapy is becoming a standard practice also in adults in order to spare the side effects of radiation and to have a second line of treatment option in case of tumour progression [2, 16, 24, 31, 35-37]. The most frequently employed agents are procarbazine, lomustine (CCNU) and vincristine (PCV) [31, 35-38]. Other chemotherapeutic agents used are carboplatin, etoposide, cisplatin, melphalan, thiotepa and other nitrosourea drugs, as well as interferon-β. Many genetic abnormalities are encountered in brain neoplasm and many of these identified may emphasize potential diagnostic, therapeutic and prognostic implications [6, 37].

Histopathology and Neurooncology

Oligodendrogliomas exhibit an infiltrative growth pattern, although not such extensive as astrocytomas [2, 7, 16, 24, 39, 40]. According to the growth pattern and histological characteristics, two types are distinguished by the WHO. The first group are diffuse or well differentiated oligodendrogliomas, designated as WHO grade II. The second group includes anaplastic oligodendrogliomas. These are the more malignant variant and therefore designated as WHO grade III [7, 21, 41]. There are 23% of anaplastic and 77% of low-grade oligodendrogliomas. Diffuse oligodendrogliomas contain cells that morphologically resemble normal oligodendroglia. They are oval to round and uniform with round nuclei, often with characteristic fried egg appearance due to perinuclear haloes formation after fixation. Cell density is moderate to low with a delicate blood vessel network among them. Occasionally, nuclear atypia and mitotic figures may be encountered, but they are mild. Microcalcification, which may be often present in the adjacent brain, is helpful in radiological diagnosis [15, 21, 39, 41, 42]. The anaplastic oligodendrogliomas, on the other hand, show focal or diffuse histological features of malignancy, including high cell density, necrosis and noticeable microvascular proliferation, marked cellular atypia and mitotic activity. They may evolve from a low-grade oligodendroglioma, becoming gradually more anaplastic over time, or present *de novo*, without a precedent low-grade lesion. Some grade III oligodendrogliomas may over time even transform to glioblastoma [2, 6, 41]. According to the tumour cell morphology, two types have been described: pure oligodendrogliomas and mixed gliomas or oligoastrocytomas, containing both neoplastic oligodendroglia and astrocytes [2, 41, 43-45].

THE IMPORTANCE OF MOLECULAR MARKERS

Oligodendrogliomas are heterogeneous tumours with a variable response to treatment. Because no specific immunohistological markers for oligodendrogliomas exist, the histological diagnosis and grading of oligodendrogliomas may be challenging for pathologists [6]. The clinical variability underlines the need for molecular markers that can reliably aid in diagnosis and also guide clinical management. About two decades ago, the first glioma-associated molecular marker was found with complete chromosome 1p and 19q co-deletion [9-11, 13, 16, 42, 46, 47]. This co-deletion is not only of diagnostic feature, but also carries prognostic information and is a predictive marker of response to chemotherapy. Molecular profiling of these tumours has identified several other markers with potential clinical significance. More recently described biomarkers include non-balanced translocation leading to 1p/19q co-deletion, mutations of the IDH1, IDH2 and CDKN2A gene, promoter hypermethylation of the MGMT gene and mutations of FUBP1 (on 1p) or CIC (on 19q). This discovery has greatly enhanced the understanding of oligodendroglioma biology and subsequently, new biomarkers have been found. Although diagnostic, their prognostic and predictive roles are at the moment less clear as all still require further validation before they may be implemented as clinical decision-making tools [15, 16, 47-50]. Various genetic markers have been described in connection to oligodendroglial tumours and are briefly discussed below.

Chromosomes 1 and 19 and the Prognostic and Diagnostic Value of 1p and 19q Abnormalities

As already stated, abnormalities in chromosomes 1 and 19 are the most significant for oligodendrogliomas. A combined loss of 1p and 19q identifies a group of good prognosis tumours and has been reported in 60% to 70%. On the other hand, the incidence of either 1p or 19q deletions is 75% [3, 6, 21, 22]. 1p and 19q losses are encountered in 80% to 90% of grade II and in 50% to 70% of grade III oligodendrogliomas [21]. On the contrary, childhood oligodendrogliomas only rarely exhibit chromosomal abnormalities. In adults, in majority of cases chromosome losses involve the entire long arm of chromosome 19 and are present in connection with losses from chromosome 1p. They were observed to be more common in frontal lobe than in temporal lobe tumours [53, 54].

Pure oligodendrogliomas show better prognosis than astrocytomas of the same grade and oligoastrocytomas are prognostically in between the former two [6]. For management of tumours and for prognostic and therapeutic decisions, it is important to identify the tumour type correctly [45]. Microscopical appearance, which forms the basis for distinction of gliomas, is not always as clear as necessary to set the diagnosis directly. It is particularly difficult to distinguish oligodendrogliomas and oligoastrocytomas. In literature studies, the diagnostic concordance observed in these tumours may range from 52% to 86% among pathologists [53]. This fact necessitated a search for an additional diagnostic tool for the oligodendrogliomas. Two factors influence the difficulties in histopathological diagnostics: I) lack of a definitive immunohistochemical cell marker in oligodendroglial tumours and II) a high variation in tumour microscopic morphology. Genetically, a combined loss of 1p and 19q is typical for oligodendrogliomas and rare in gliomas of other type, while isolated 19q loss occurs in mixed oligoastrocytomas and in astrocytomas [53-55]. Chromosome 1p and 19q status may be assessed by a variety of techniques, such as microsatellite analysis, fluorescence in situ hybridization, genomic hybridization, loss of heterozygosity studies and quantitative polymerase chain reactions [21, 53, 55].

Because the 1p and 19q deletion in combination with histological features are predictive factors of tumour response principally to chemotherapy and to radiotherapy as well, many centres are taking the advantage of 1p and 19q status as a laboratory test. This is used in conjunction to clinical status, imaging and patohistological features for predicting patient response to treatment [53, 56-58]. It enables tailoring the most effective and appropriate therapy for the individual patient [45, 55, 59]. Oliogodendrogliomas harbouring 1p and 19q deletion behave more indolently and respond favourably to procarbazine, lomustine and vincristine (PCV) chemotherapy and temozolomide as well as to radiotherapy [55, 60]. For example, the reported correlation between 1p and 19q loss and PCV regimen in treatment response ranged from 93% to 100%. Temozolomide as a replacement for PCV therapy, due to a better toxicity profile, showed 46% to 55% response rate to treatment. Also time to progression of the disease correlated with 1p and 19q loss [6, 56, 59]. On the other hand, the therapeutic sensitivity of 1p and 19q-intact tumours is less favourable and survival is therefore shorter [57-59].

Besides being a valuable diagnostic marker due to its specificity, it was discovered that 1p and 19q loss also acts as a powerful marker in prognosis of the disease and as a predictor of chemotherapeutic response and survival [53, 55, 60]. However, there are still unexplained issues in connection to 1p and 19q loss. To begin with, the genes and their exact functions in the pathogenesis of oligodendrogliomas, located on the long arms of chromosomes 1 and 19, need to be identified and some patients with 1p and 19q intact tumours respond well to therapy and vice versa [6,59]. Despite the fact that 1p and 19q status helps in selecting patients with respect to therapeutic regimen, there were no revolutionary improvements in the treatment outcomes [55]. Further investigation is required in order to elucidate the unsolved questions in oligodendroglioma biology.

MGMT Mutation

Another factor reported to bear prognostic significance is o6-methylguanine-DNAmethyltransferase (MGMT), an enzyme involved in DNA repair [61, 62]. In many tumours, including gliomas, alterations in DNA may be found, such as methylation of the promoter region and their genes. Hypermethylated DNA is less readily accessible to transcription factors and results in loss of gene function. As MGMT is one of the key factors in resistance to chemotherapy, hypermethylation inhibits the repair mechanism due to a lower level of the active enzyme [6, 21, 59, 62]. MGMT methylation rates in oligodendrogliomas range from 25% to 85% and were reported to be strongly associated with 1p and 19q loss [56, 59]. However, response rate to chemotherapy and time to progression of oligodendrogliomas were not observed to be in correlation with the degree of MGMT methylation, as is the case with glioblastoma, where promoter methylation correlated with response to alkylating agent treatment and survival. The cause probably lies in different genes and patterns of promoter methylation, which is present in astrocytic cells [21, 59, 61-63].

Hypermethylation

Another common finding in oligodendrogliomas is hypermethylation of DNA regions that code for MGMT genes. The end result is transcriptional silencing of genes responsible for DNA repair enzyme, which may contribute to higher chemosensitivity [21, 54].

Mutations in p53Gene

Mutations in p53 gene are described in 10% to 15% of tumours without 1p and 19q loss [21]. Such tumours arise most commonly in the temporal lobes; histologically they are anaplastic or mixed oligodendrogliomas and express poor chemosensitivity [64, 65]. Chemotherapy response rate was observed only in 33% of patients with p53 mutation and intact 1p and 19q chromosomes, as opposed to tumours with intact p53 gene and 1p and 19q or only 1p mutation, where the response rate was 100% [21, 64].

Growth Factors and Other Genetic Abnormalities

Growth factors overexpression includes epidermal growth factor receptor (EGFR), vascular endothelial growth factor (VEGF) and platelet-derived growth factor (PDGF) [21, 66]. EGFR overexpression was observed in 50% of oligodendrogliomas; the percentage of other two overexpressed factors is somewhat lower. Other chromosomal abnormalities consist of genetic abnormalities or losses from chromosomes 10q and 9p. They are preferentially encountered in anaplastic oligiodendrogliomas without of 1p and 19q loss [21, 53]. Additionally, oligodendrocyte transcription factors, such as Olig 1 and Olig 2 that may be used as specific markers, are highly expressed in oligodendrogliomas, as well as in astrocytomas [21, 67, 68].

CONCLUSION

Oligodendroglial tumours with 1p and 19q loss demonstrate a better overall prognosis due to more indolent clinical behaviour and higher sensitivity to treatment. The 1p and 19q status acts as a prognostic marker, since its loss is associated with an improved outcome compared to non-1p and 19q deleted oligodendrogliomas and astrocytomas of a similar grade [56-59].

1p and 19q testing proved to be particularly useful for determining the tumour type in morphologically ambiguous cases, as it acts as a valid marker of classical oligodendroglial tumours. Additionally, 1p and 19q loss is a marker of clinical utility, helping to assess tumour sensitivity to chemotherapy and harbouring the potential for improving the diagnosis and survival of oligodendroglioma patients as well as future clinical practice [55-58].

REFERENCES

[1] Giampaoli S. Epidemiology of major age-related diseases in women compared to men. *Aging (Milano)* 2000; 12: 93-105.

[2] Engelhard HH, Stelea A, Mundt A. Oligodendroglioma and anaplastic oligodendroglioma: clinical features, treatment and prognosis. *Surg. Neurol.* 2003; 60: 443-56.

[3] Pytel P, Lukas RV. Update on diagnosic practice: tumors of the nervous system. *Arch. Pathol. Lab. Med.* 2009; 133: 1062-77.

[4] Gilbert MR, Lang FF. Management of patients with low-grade gliomas. *Neurol. Clin.* 2007; 25: 1073-88.

[5] Asthagiri AR, Pouratian N, Sherman J, Ahmed G, Shaffrey ME. Advances in brain tumor surgery. *Neurol. Clin.* 2007; 25: 975-1003.

[6] van den Bent MJ, Reni M, Gatta G, Vecht C. Oligodendroglioma. *Crit. Rev. Oncol. Hematol.* 2008; 66: 262-72.

[7] Komori T. Pathology and Genetics of Diffuse Gliomas in Adults. *Neurol. Med. Chir. (Tokyo)* 2015; 55: 28-37.

[8] Simonetti G, Gaviani P, Botturi A, Innocenti A, Lamperti E, Silvani A. Clinical management of grade III oligodendroglioma. *Cancer Manag. Res.* 2015; 7: 213-23.

[9] Appin CL, Brat DJ. Molecular pathways in gliomagenesis and their relevance to neuropathologic diagnosis. *Adv. Anat. Pathol.* 2015; 22: 50-8.

[10] Appin CL, Brat DJ. Molecular genetics of gliomas. *Cancer J.* 2014; 20: 66-72.

[11] Speirs CK, Simpson JR, Robinson CG, DeWees TA, Tran DD, Linette G, Chicoine MR, Dacey RG, Rich KM, Dowling JL, Leuthardt EC, Zipfel GJ, Kim AH, Huang J. Impact of 1p/19q codeletion and histology on outcomes of anaplastic gliomas treated with radiation therapy and temozolomide. *Int. J. Radiat. Oncol. Biol. Phys.* 2015; 91: 268-76.

[12] Khan KA, Abbasi AN, Ali N. Treatment updates regarding anaplastic oligodendroglioma and anaplastic oligoastrocytoma. *J. Coll. Physicians Surg. Pak.* 2014; 24: 935-9.

[13] Brandner S, von Deimling A. Diagnostic, prognostic and predictive relevance of molecular markers in gliomas. *Neuropathol. Appl. Neurobiol.* 2015; 41: 694-720.

[14] Siker ML, Chakravarti A, Mehta MP. Should concomitant and adjuvant treatment with temozolomide be used as standard therapy in patients with anaplastic glioma? *Crit. Rev. Oncol. Hematol.* 2006; 60: 99-111.

[15] Wrensch M, Minn Y, Chew T, Bondy M, Berger MS. Epidemiology of primary brain tumors: current concepts and review of the literature. *Neuro Oncol. 2002*; 4: 278-99.

[16] Chowdhary S, Chamberlain MC. Oligodendroglial tumors. *Expert Rev. Neurother* 2006; 6: 519-32.

[17] Ohgaki H Epidemiology of brain tumors. *Methods Mol. Biol.* 2009; 472: 323-42.

[18] van den Bent MJ. Diagnosis and management of oligodendroglioma. *Semin. Oncol.* 2004; 31: 645-52.

[19] Wrensch M, Fisher JL, Schwartzbaum JA, Bondy M, Berger M, Aldape KD. The molecular epidemiology of gliomas in adults. *Neurosurg. Focus* 2005; 19: E5.

[20] Cairncross G, Macdonald D, Ludwin S. Chemotherapy for anaplastic oligodendroglioma. *J. Clin. Oncol.* 1994; 12: 2013-21.

[21] Hilton DA, Melling C. Genetic markers in teh assesment of intrinsic brain tumours. *Current Diagnostic Pathology* 2004; 10: 83-92.

[22] Scelsi R. Epidemiology of cerebral gliomas. *Minerva Med.* 1984; 75: 1259-63.

[23] Cairncross JG, Ueki K, Zlatescu MC. Specific genetic predictors of chemotherapeutic response and survival in patients with anaplastic oligodendrogliomas. *J. Natl. Cancer Inst.* 1998; 90: 1473-9.

[24] Jaeckle KA. Oligodendroglial tumors. *Semin Oncol* 2014; 41: 468-77.

[25] Liigant A, Haldre S, Oun A, Linnamägi U, Saar A, Asser T, Kaasik AE. Seizure disorders in patients with brain tumors. *Eur. Neurol.* 2001; 45: 46-51.

[26] Engelhard HH. Current diagnosis and treatment of oligodendroglioma. *Neurosurg. Focus* 2002; 12: E2.

[27] Celli P, Nofrone I, Palma L, Cantore G, Fortuna A. Cerebral oligodendroglioma: prognostic factors and life history. *Neurosurgery* 1994; 35: 1018-35.

[28] Zustovich F, Della Puppa A, Scienza R, Anselmi P, Furlan C, Cartei G. Metastatic oligodendrogliomas: a review of the literature and case report. *Acta Neurochir (Wien)* 2008; 150: 699-703.

[29] Volavsek M, Lamovec J, Popović M. Extraneural metastases of anaplastic oligodendroglial tumors. *Pathol. Res. Pract.* 2009; 205: 502-7.

[30] Burton EC, Prados MD. Malignant gliomas. *Curr. Treat Options Oncol.* 2000; 1: 459-68.

[31] Bromberg JE, van den Bent MJ. Oligodendrogliomas: molecular biology and treatment. *Oncologist* 2009; 14: 155-63.

[32] Gannett DE, Wisbeck WM, Silbergeld DL, Berger MS. The role of postoperative irradiation in the treatment of oligodendroglioma. *Int. J. Radiat. Oncol. Biol. Phys.* 1994; 30: 567-73.

[33] Paleologos NA, Cairncross JG. Treatment of oligodendroglioma: an update. *Neuro. Oncol.* 1999; 1: 61-8.

[34] Bullard DE, Rawlings CE 3rd, Phillips B, Cox EB, Schold SC Jr, Burger P, Halperin EC. Oligodendroglioma. An analysis of the value of radiation therapy. *Cancer* 1987; 60: 2179-88.

[35] van den Bent MJ. Chemotherapy of oligodendroglial tumours: current developments. *Forum (Genova)* 2000; 10: 108-18.

[36] van den Bent MJ. New perspectives for the diagnosis and treatment of oligodendrogliomav. *Expert Rev. Anticancer Ther.* 2001; 1: 348-56.

[37] Soffietti R. Chemotherapy of anaplastic oligodendroglial tumours. *Expert Opin. Pharmacother* 2004; 5: 295-306.

[38] Medical Research Council Brain Tumor Working Party. Randomized trial of procarbazine, lomustine, and vincristine in the adjuvant treatment of high-grade astrocytoma: a Medical Research Council trial. *J. Clin. Oncol.* 2001; 19: 509-18.

[39] Louis DN. Molecular pathology of malignant gliomas. *Annu. Rev. Pathol.* 2006; 1:.97-117.

[40] Wong ET, Hess KR, Gleason MJ, Jaeckle KA, Kyritsis AP, Prados MD, Levin VA, Yung WK. Outcomes and prognostic factors in recurrent glioma patients enrolled onto phase II clinical trials. *J. Clin. Oncol.* 1999; 17: 2572-8.

[41] Engelhard HH, Stelea A, Cochran EJ. Oligodendroglioma: pathology and molecular biology. *Surg. Neurol.* 2002; 58: 111-7.

[42] Wesseling P, van den Bent M, Perry A. Oligodendroglioma: pathology, molecular mechanisms and markers. *Acta Neuropathol.* 2015; 129: 809-27.

[43] van den Bent MJ. Anaplastic oligodendroglioma and oligoastrocytoma. *Neurol. Clin.* 2007; 25: 1089-109.
[44] Engelhard HH, Stelea A, Mundt A. Oligodendroglioma and anaplastic oligodendroglioma: clinical features, treatment, and prognosis. *Surg. Neurol.* 2003; 60: 443-56.
[45] Figarella-Branger D, Colin C, Coulibaly B, Quilichini B, Maues De Paula A, Fernandez C, Bouvier C. Histological and molecular classification of gliomas. *Rev. Neurol. (Paris)* 2008; 164: 505-15.
[46] Appin CL, Brat DJ. Biomarker-driven diagnosis of diffuse gliomas. *Mol. Aspects Med.* 2015. [Epub ahead of print]
[47] Siegal T. Clinical impact of molecular biomarkers in gliomas. *J. Clin. Neurosci.* 2015; 22: 437-44.
[48] Sahebjam S, McNamara MG, Mason WP. Emerging biomarkers in anaplastic oligodendroglioma: implications for clinical investigation and patient management. *CNS Oncol.* 2013; 2: 351-8.
[49] Hofer S, Rushing E, Preusser M, Marosi C. Molecular biology of high-grade gliomas: what should the clinician know? *Chin. J. Cancer* 2014; 33: 4-7.
[50] Sahm F, Koelsche C, Meyer J, Pusch S, Lindenberg K, Mueller W, Herold-Mende C, von Deimling A, Hartmann C. CIC and FUBP1 mutations in oligodendrogliomas, oligoastrocytomas and astrocytomas. *Acta Neuropathol.* 2012; 123: 853-60.
[51] Bromberg JE, van den Bent MJ. Oligodendrogliomas: molecular biology *and treatment Oncologist* 2009; 14: 155-63.
[52] van den Bent MJ. Diagnosis and management of oligodendroglioma. *Semin. Oncol.* 2004; 31: 645-52.
[53] Gadji M, Fortin D, Tsanaclis AM, Drouin R. Is the 1p/19q deletion a diagnostic marker of oligodendrogliomas? *Cancer Genet Cytogenet* 2009; 194: 12-22.
[54] Stupp R, Hegi ME. Neuro-oncology: oligodendroglioma and molecular markers. *Lancet Neurol* 2007; 6: 10-2.
[55] Aldape K, Burger PC, Perry A. Clinicopathologic aspects of 1p/19q loss and the diagnosis of oligodendroglioma. *Arch. Pathol. Lab. Med.* 2007; 131: 242-51.
[56] Idbaih A, Omuro A, Ducray F, Hoang-Xuan K. Molecular genetic markers as predictors of response to chemotherapy in gliomas. *Curr. Opin. Oncol.* 2007; 19: 606-11.
[57] Fontaine D, Vandenbos F, Lebrun C, Paquis V, Frenay M. Diagnostic and prognostic values of 1p and 19q deletions in adult gliomas: critical

review of the literature and implications in daily clinical practice. *Rev. Neurol. (Paris)* 2008; 164: 595-604.

[58] Sonabend AM, Lesniak MS. Oligodendrogliomas: clinical significance of 1p and 19q chromosomal deletions. *Expert Rev. Neurother* 2005; 5: S25-32.

[59] Brandes AA, Tosoni A, Cavallo G, Reni M, Franceschi E, Bonaldi L, Bertorelle R, Gardiman M, Ghimenton C, Iuzzolino P, Pession A, Blatt V, Ermani M. Correlations between O6-methylguanine DNA methyltransferase promoter methylation status, 1p and 19q deletions, and response to temozolomide in anaplastic and recurrent oligodendroglioma: a prospective GICNO study. *J. Clin. Oncol.* 2006; 24: 4746-53.

[60] Michotte A, Chaskis C, Sadones J, Veld PI, Neyns B. Primary leptomeningeal anaplastic oligodendroglioma with a 1p36-19q13 deletion: Report of a unique case successfully treated with Temozolomide. *J. Neurol. Sci.* 2009 [Epub ahead of print].

[61] Cankovic M, Mikkelsen T, Rosenblum ML, Zarbo RJ. A simplified laboratory validated assay for MGMT promoter hypermethylation analysis of glioma specimens from formalin-fixed paraffin-embedded tissue. *Lab. Invest* 2007; 87: 392-7.

[62] Mueller WC, von Deimling A. Gene regulation by methylation. *Recent Results Cancer Res.* 2009; 171: 217-39.

[63] Norden AD, Wen PY. Glioma therapy in adults. *Neurologist* 2006; 12: 279-92.

[64] Ino Y, Betensky RA, Zlatescu MC, Sasaki H, Macdonald DR, Stemmer-Rachamimov AO, Ramsay DA, Cairncross JG, Louis DN. Molecular subtypes of anaplastic oligodendroglioma: implications for patient management at diagnosis. *Clin. Cancer Res.* 2001; 7: 839-45.

[65] Mueller W, Hartmann C, Hoffmann A, Lanksch W, Kiwit J, Tonn J, Veelken J, Schramm J, Weller M, Wiestler OD, Louis DN, von Deimling A. Genetic signature of oligoastrocytomas correlates with tumor location and denotes distinct molecular subsets. *Am. J. Pathol.* 2002; 161: 313-9.

[66] Ducray F, Idbaih A, de Reyniès A, Bièche I, Thillet J, Mokhtari K, Lair S, Marie Y, Paris S, Vidaud M, Hoang-Xuan K, Delattre O, Delattre JY, Sanson M. Anaplastic oligodendrogliomas with 1p19q codeletion have a proneural gene expression profile. *Mol. Cancer* 2008; 7: 41.

[67] Riemenschneider MJ, Koy TH, Reifenberger G. Expression of oligodendrocyte lineage genes in oligodendroglial and astrocytic gliomas. *Acta Neuropathol.* 2004; 107: 277-82.

[68] Li H, Lu Y, Smith HK, Richardson WD. Olig1 and Sox10 interact synergistically to drive myelin basic protein transcription in oligodendrocytes. *J. Neurosci.* 2007; 27: 14375-82.

In: Oligodendrogliomas (ODs)
Editor: Chad Reeves
ISBN: 978-1-63484-278-5

Chapter 3

OLIGODENDROGLIOMA LOOK-ALIKES: THE HISTOPATHOLOGIC DIFFERENTIAL DIAGNOSIS

Richard A. Prayson**, MD, MEd
Department of Anatomic Pathology
Cleveland Clinic, Cleveland, Ohio, US

ABSTRACT

In the era of molecular pathology, oligodendrogliomas have emerged as a distinctive subgroup of gliomas. Recognition of the presence of large deletions on chromosomes 1p and 19q and the correlation of these deletions with chemoresponsiveness has had significant impact on the clinical management of these tumors and on prognosis. Some people have even gone so far as to propose that these deletions should be required to make a definitive diagnosis. The classic histologic appearance of these tumors is also somewhat distinctive – cells with rounded nuclei, absent nucleoli, scant cytoplasm and pericellular clearing (so-called fried egg appearance). From a purely morphologic perspective, however, there are a variety of other neoplasms which may have a similar appearance (look-alikes) and can potentially result in diagnostic confusion or misdiagnosis. The focus of this chapter is to examine the histopathologic differential

* Correspondence: Richard Prayson, MD, Med, Department of Anatomic Pathology, L25, Cleveland Clinic, Cleveland, OH 44195 USA, Phone: 216-444-8805, Fax: 216-445-6967, Email: praysor@ccf.org.

diagnoses of oligodendroglioma and discuss features one can employ to sort through these differentials. Among the lesions to be discussed include astrocytomas and mixed gliomas, dysembryoplastic neuroepithelial tumors, neurocytomas, clear cell ependymomas, lymphomas, and pilocytic astrocytomas.

INTRODUCTION

Oligodendrogliomas have been long recognized as a distinct glioma type. They have a characteristic histologic phenotype, a recognized genetic signature, and a biologic behavior that affords patients with these tumors a generally better prognosis and an increased likelihood of responsiveness to chemotherapy, as compared with the more common diffuse or fibrillary astrocytomas. For treatment and prognosis reasons, arriving at a correct histopathologic diagnosis when examining tumors which have been biopsied or resected is critically important in ensuring optimal clinical management. The focus of this chapter is to examine the histopathologic features of oligodendrogliomas and of an assortment of other central nervous system neoplasms that can resemble them and review features that allow one to sort through these histopathologic differential diagnoses.

WHAT DOES OLIGODENDROGLIOMA LOOK LIKE?

Normal white matter (Figure 1) is marked by a predominant population of small cells with rounded nuclei, vesicular chromatin and scant cytoplasm which represent oligodendrocytes [1]. These cells are primarily responsible for maintaining myelin around axonal processes which transverse the white matter. Intermixed with these cells are astrocytes, microglia and the endothelial cells lining small caliber blood vessels.

Oligodendrogliomas are generally marked by a predominant cell population resembling oligodendrocytes [2] (Figure 2). These cells generally have rounded nuclei, no nucleoli and scant cytoplasm. In low grade tumors, there is typically no more than mild nuclear pleomorphism. In formalin-fixed sections, pericellular clearing or a halo (fried-egg appearance) may be evident. This is an artifact that is the result of delayed formalin fixation and is not evident in rapidly fixed tissue sections or on frozen section. Because the tumor cells contain little cytoplasm and are process poor, the tumor's arcuate capillary vasculature or "chicken wire" vasculature usually stands out (Figure 3). The majority of tumors demonstate foci of calcification (Figure 4).

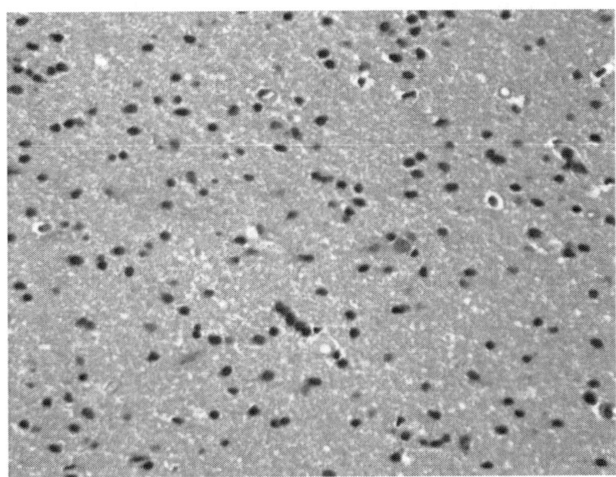

Figure 1. White matter is comprised primarily of small rounded cells (oligodendrocytes), occasional astrocytes (larger cell), and small capillaries (hematoxylin and eosin, original magnification 400X).

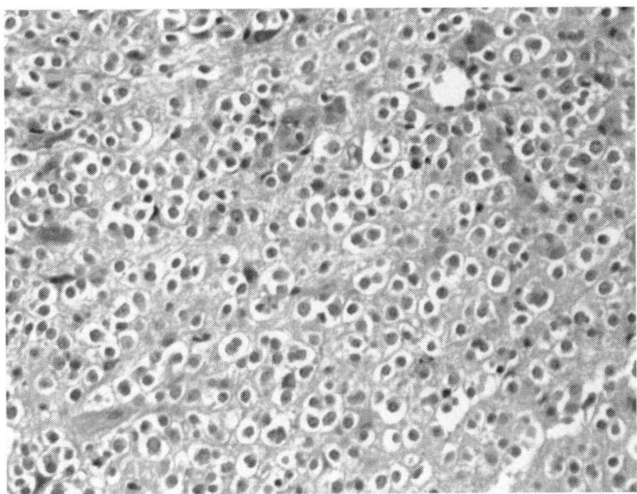

Figure 2. A low grade oligodendroglioma marked by a monomorphic proliferation of rounded cells resembling oligodendrocytes (hematoxylin and eosin, original magnification 400X).

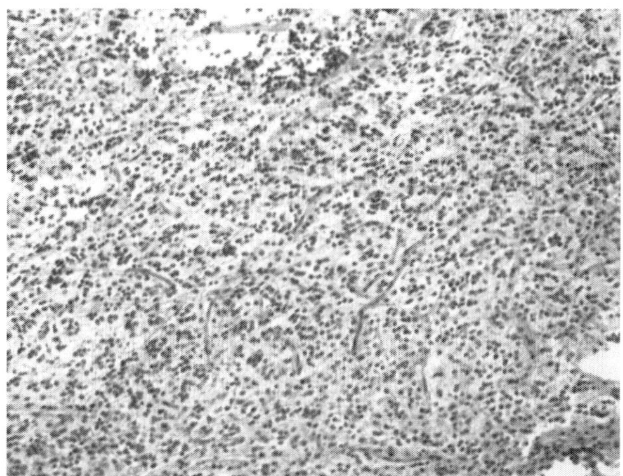

Figure 3. An arcuate capillary vasculature in oligodendroglioma is often readily discernible (hematoxylin and eosin, original magnification 200X).

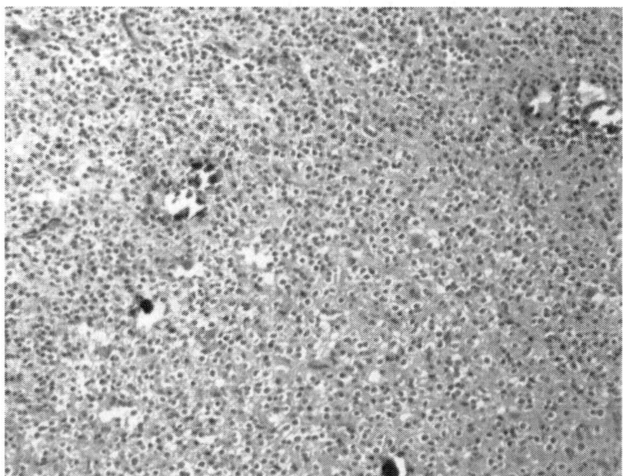

Figure 4. Dystrophic mineralization is frequently observed in oligodendrogliomas (hematoxylin and eosin, original magnification 400X).

Areas of microcystic degeneration may be present in some tumors (Figure 5). Oligodendrogliomas typically arise in the white matter and are by nature infiltrative neoplasms. Commonly, tumor cells can be seen infiltrating through contiguous gray matter tissues. Cells frequently can be seen satelliting around preexistent structures such as neurons and blood vessels and may be seen aggregating at the surface of the brain (subpial aggregation) (Figure 6). Extension into the leptomeninges is not common. Some tumors have prominent numbers of gemistocytic-like cells with more abundant eosinophilic cytoplasm and eccentrically placed oligodendendroglial-like nuclei (Figure 7). These so-called minigemistocytes do not carry any prognostic significance but may result in an erroneous diagnosis of gemistocytic astrocytoma, if their presence is misinterpreted.

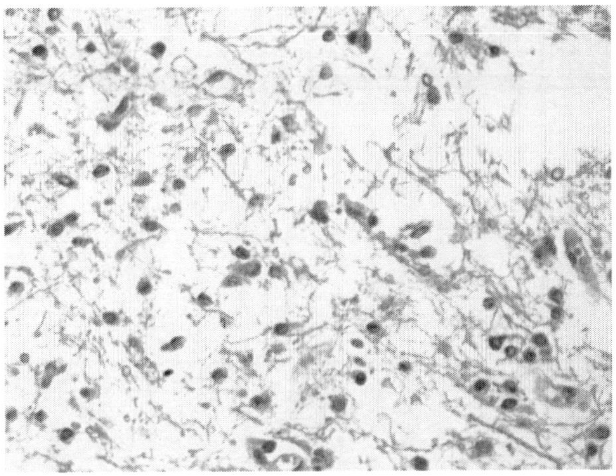

Figure 5. Microcystic changes may be focally present in oligodendrogliomas (hematoxylin and eosin, original magnification 400X).

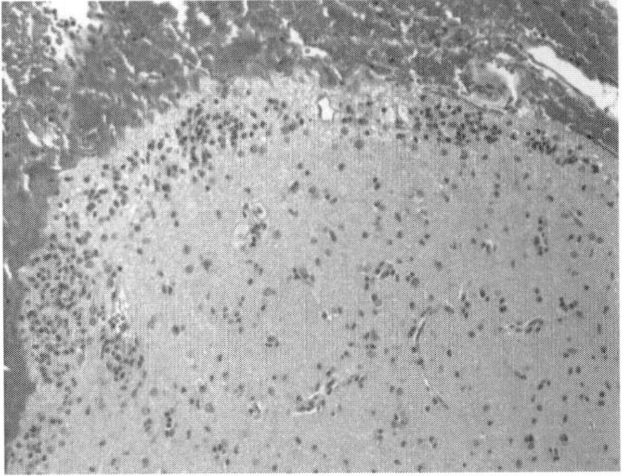

Figure 6. Oligodendrogliomas are infiltrative neoplasms. Frequently, tumor cells are seen in the cortex and aggregating under the surface of the brain (subpial aggregation) (hematoxylin and eosin, original magnification 200X).

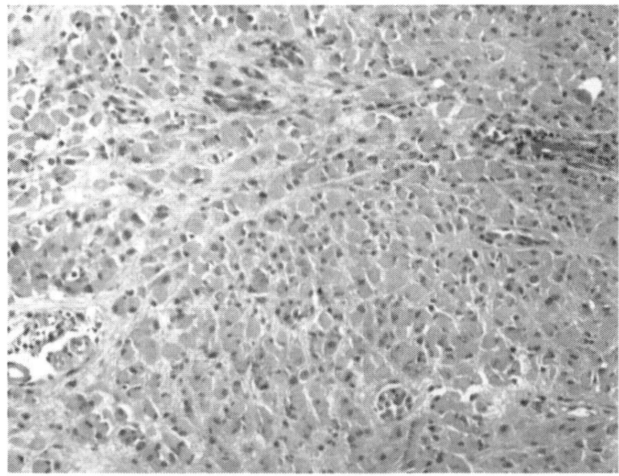

Figure 7. An area of oligodendroglioma marked by larger, eosinophilic cells known as minigemistocytes (hematoxylin and eosin, original magnification 200X).

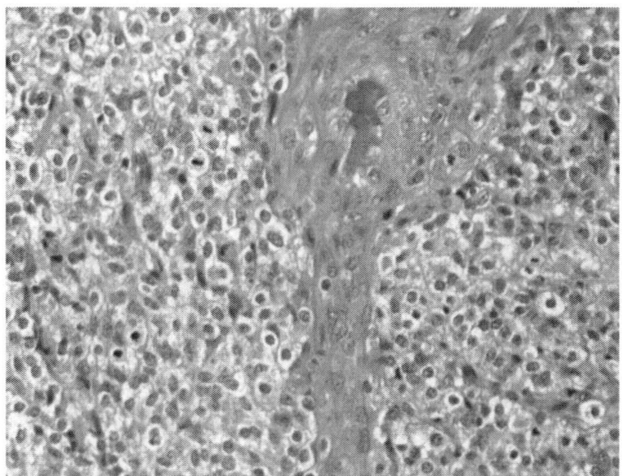

Figure 8. An anaplastic oligodendroglioma marked by increased numbers of mitotic figures and vascular proliferative changes (hematoxylin and eosin, original magnification 400X).

The World Health Organization (WHO) classification of brain tumors, stratifies oligodendrogliomas into low grade (WHO grade II) and high grade (WHO grade III) lesions [3]. The parameters that are used to assess tumor grade include cellularity and degree of atypia, mitotic activity, vascular proliferative changes and necrosis (Figures 8 and 9). These are similar parameters to what is used in grading the diffuse or fibrillary astrocytomas;

however, the thresholds for designating a tumor as high grade are different. In general, tumors with increased mitoses, on the order of 5 or 6 per 10 high power fields, increased cellularity and vascular proliferative changes and/or necrosis warrant a diagnosis of anaplastic oligodendroglioma. Necrosis does not equate with a diagnosis of glioblastoma or grade IV glioma in these cases.

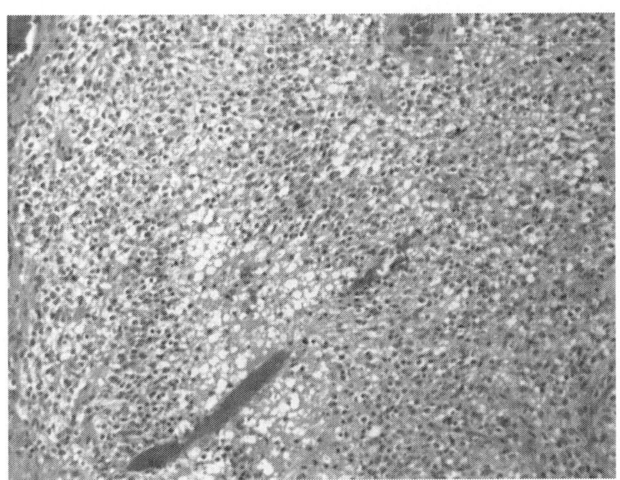

Figure 9. An anaplastic oligodendroglioma characterized by an area of geographic necrosis (hematoxylin and eosin, original magnification 200X).

Rates of cell proliferation, as evidenced by immunomarkers of proliferation such as Ki-67 and MIB-1, tend to be generally greater in high grade lesions than low grade lesions [3-5]. There can be considerable tumor heterogeneity, though, with respect to immunostaining with cell proliferation markers (Figures 10 and 11). By convention, the area of tumor with the most proliferation is used to determine the labeling index. There is considerable overlap in terms of reported labeling index ranges between low grade and anaplastic tumors such that indices are not practically useful in most cases for grade determination (unless it is very high).

Oligodendrogliomas, from an immunohistochemistry standpoint, do not have a distinctive phenotype [2]. Part of the struggle has been the fact that the cell cytoplasm is rather scant and nondescript which has made finding unique features or proteins to target for immunostaining a challenge. Olig 2 stains the nuclei of oligodendrogliomas but can also stain many astrocytomas. Minigemistocytes with increased cytoplasm are often highlighted with GFAP (glial fibrillary acidic protein) and S-100 protein antibodies, but again, this is nonspecific. Antibodies for neuronal markers such as NeuN, synaptophysin and neurofilament protein may be focally present in a subset of tumors.

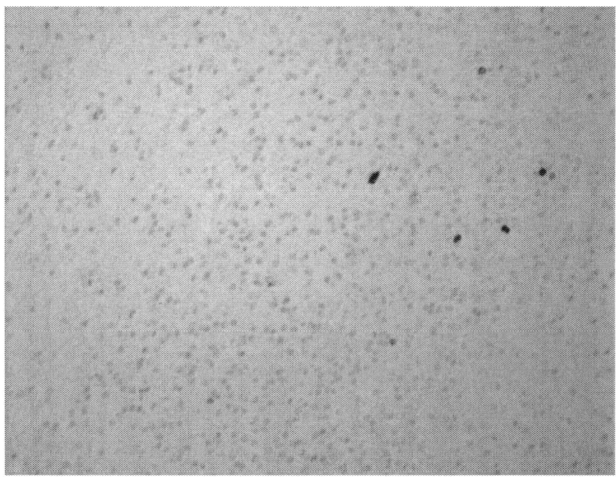

Figure 10. Ki-67 immunostaining in a low grade oligodendroglioma showing rare tumor cell positivity (original magnification 400X).

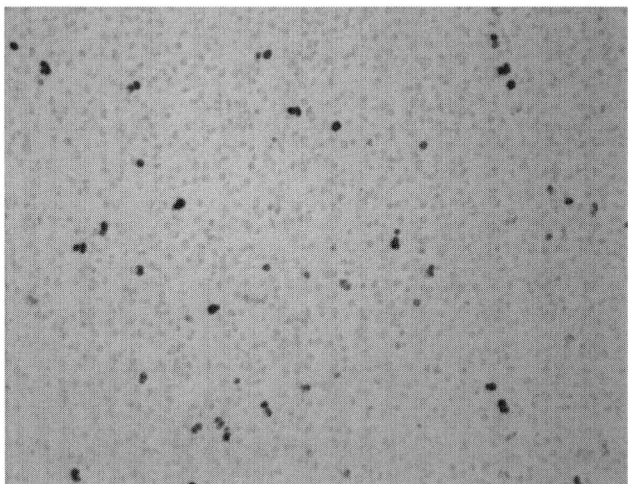

Figure 11. Ki-67 immunostaining in the same low grade oligodendroglioma as in Figure 10. This high power field is contiguous with the high power field photographed in Figure 10 and highlights the regional heterogeneity of these tumors (original magnification 400X).

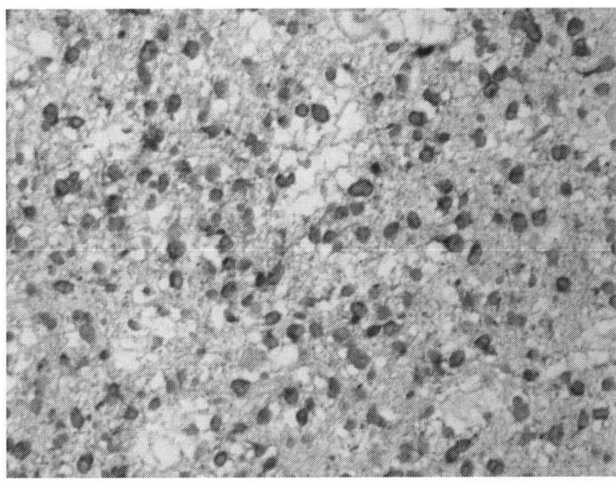

Figure 12. IDH-1 (R132H) immunostaining typically demonstrates diffuse positivity in the majority of oligodendrogliomas (original magnification 400X).

Molecular markers which have been more recently developed have proven to be potentially more useful. Extensive p53 immunostaining is unusual in classic oligodendrogliomas and is a feature more commonly encountered in a subset of diffuse astrocytomas [6-8]. Most oligodendrogliomas demonstrate widespread IDH-1(R132H) immunoreactivity [9-10] (Figure 12). ATRX mutations resulting in a loss of ATRX staining is not a feature of these tumors; loss of staining may be seen in a subset of diffuse astrocytomas and may be useful in the differentiating oligodendrogliomas from some astrocytomas [11-12]. Chromosome 1p and 19q codeletion appears to be very characteristic of most oligodendrogliomas and will generally not be evident in all of the lesions in its differential diagnosis [10, 13]. Some people have gone on to suggest that these characteristic large chromosomal deletions are part of the definition of these tumors.

Diffuse Astrocytoma versus Oligodendroglioma

Perhaps the most common tumor to arise in the histologic differential diagnosis of oligodendroglioma is astrocytoma. Diffuse or fibrillary astroctyomas are the most common primary tumors of the central nervous system. Distinction between the two tumor types is important from therapeutic and prognostic standpoints. Grade for grade, astrocytomas tend to behave in a more aggressive fashion. Oligodendrogliomas with the signature chromosome 1p and 19q deletions respond well to certain types of chemotherapy in contrast to astrocytomas which generally do not respond as well to the same chemotherapy. Both tumors may present in a similar fashion and may look similar on imaging studies.

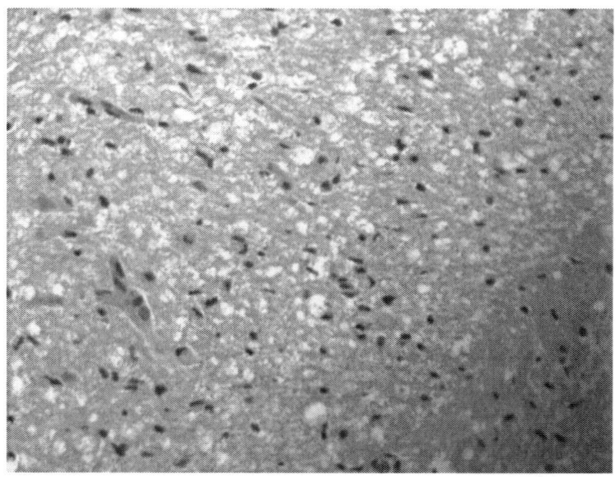

Figure 13. A low grade diffuse astrocytoma (WHO grade II) marked by mild hypercellularity and atypical appearing astrocytic cells with nuclear pleomorphism and hyperchromasia (hematoxylin and eosin, original magnification 400X).

Histologically, astrocytomas, like oligodendrogliomas, tend to be infiltrative neoplasms without circumscript borders [2]. In contrast, neoplastic astrocytic cells tend to have more irregularly shaped nuclei in contrast to the more rounded nuclei of oligodendrogliomas (Figure 13). Nuclei tend to be enlarged and hyperchromatic. Cells often are marked by a high nuclear to cytoplasmic ratio. Tumor cells generally stain with antibody to glial fibrillary acidic protein (GFAP) and S-100 protein. A subset of tumors demonstrate isocitrate dehydrogenase [IDH-1 (R132]) immunoreactivity and a subset of tumors demonstrate loss of ATRX staining (most oligodendrogliomas, remember, are positive for both) [9-12]. Chromosomes 1p and 19q losses are generally absent in most astrocytomas, although occasional tumors may demonstrate smaller deletions on one or the other chromosome; the clinical significance of these findings is not agreed upon in the literature [14-15]. Loss of heterozygosity (LOH) on chromosome 10q is present in a majority of astrocytomas [16]. p53 mutations are rare in oligodendrogliomas and are present in a subset of astrocytomas , most notably the secondary tumors that appear to start as low grade lesions and progress to glioblastoma over time. Epidermal growth factor receptor (EGFR) amplification or overexpression is more common in an astrocytomas, especially in the primary glioblastomas and in certain variants such as the small cell variant [17]. O(6)-methylguanine-DNA-methyltransferase (MGMT) methylation abnormalities are also more frequently encountered in astrocytomas [18-20].

Like oligodendrogliomas, astrocytomas are stratified into grades according the presence or absence of certain histologic parameters. The same morphologic features are used to grade diffuse or fibrillary astrocytomas as oligodendrogliomas; however, the thresholds or criteria for assigning grade are a bit different. Unlike oligodendrogliomas, astrocytomas have a grade IV designation (glioblastoma), predicated on the presence of either necrosis or vascular proliferative changes. The presence of fewer mitotic figures is required to elevate a tumor from grade II to grade III in astrocytomas.

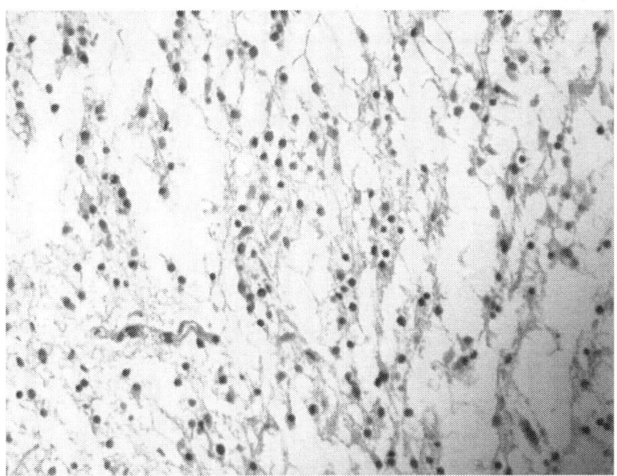

Figure 14. A rare protoplasmic astrocytoma characterized by rounded astrocytic cells with scant cytoplasm arranged against a microcystic background (hematoxylin and eosin, original magnification 400X).

A few particular variants of astrocytoma can present particular challenges in terms of differential diagnosis. The rare low grade protoplasmic astrocytoma is comprised of neoplastic astrocytes with scant cytoplasm (and subsequently scant GFAP immunoreactivity) and generally rounded nuclei [21-22] (Figure 14). The tumor cells are often arranged against a microcystic background. Tumors have been reported to more commonly arise in the frontotemporal region and generally have low rates of cell proliferation, as evidenced by Ki-67 or MIB-1 immunoreactivity; chromosome 1p deletions are not observed in these tumors.

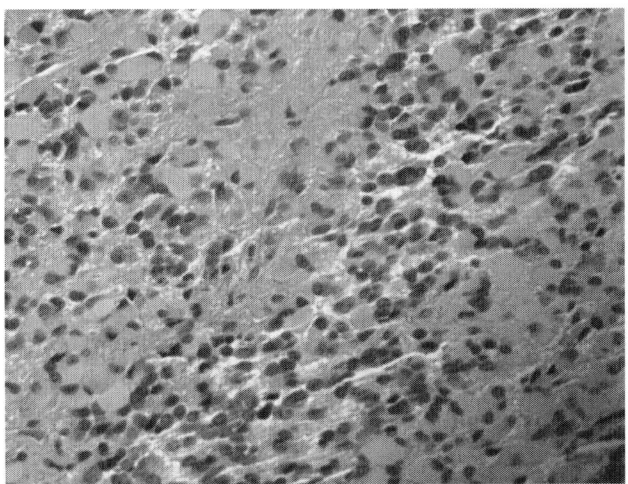

Figure 15. This gemistocytic astrocytoma is marked by an increased number of large cells with abundant eosinophilic cytoplasm (gemistocytes). Note that there is a second population of tumor cells with high nuclear to cytoplasmic ratios and elongated nuclear contours (hematoxylin and eosin, original magnification 400X).

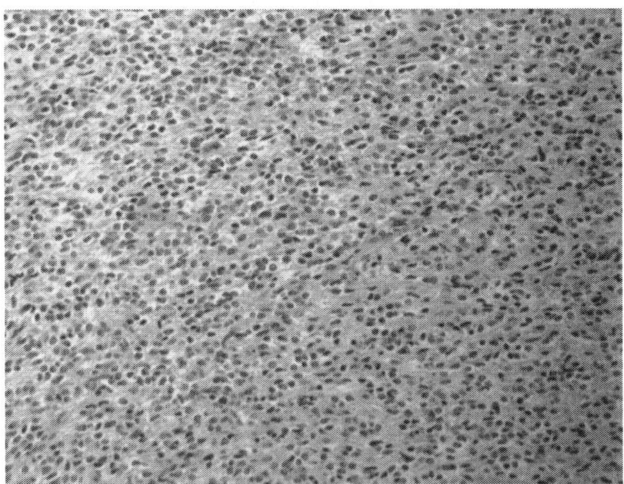

Figure 16. A subset of diffuse astrocytomas is characterized by a proliferation of generally rounded cells with scant cytoplasm, representing small cell astrocytomas (hematoxylin and eosin, original magnification 200X).

Gemistocytic astrocytomas are marked by an increased number of large astrocytic cells with abundant eosinophilic cytoplasm and eccentrically placed, irregular shaped nuclei [2] (Figure 15). Confusion of this variant with the minigemistocytic changes that may occur in an oligodendroglioma may occur. In both cases, there is usually a second population of cells in the tumor which consists of cells that look more typical of the tumor type. Gemistocytic astrocytomas tend to behave in an even more aggressive fashion than their regular astrocytoma counterparts, grade for grade.

The small cell variant of a glioblastoma can be diagnostically challenging to distinguish from an anaplastic oligodendroglioma [2] (Figure 16). Small cell astrocytomas tend to be similarly characterized by high cellular density regions with cells that do not appear as cohesive as in anaplastic oligodendrogliomas. These astrocytomas generally have nuclei with dispersed chromatin and indistinct nucleoli in contrast to the distinct nucleoli of an anaplastic oligodendroglioma. In the absence of areas that resemble more conventional appearing oligodendroglioma or astrocytoma and given the subtle nature of the histologic differences, molecular testing is often needed to more definitively distinguish the two. IDH-1 immunoreactivity is typically absent in small cell astrocytomas. Chromosome 1p and 19q deletions are not seen in the astrocytomas. EGFR amplification or overexpression is almost always present in this variant of astrocytoma.

Oligoastrocytoma/Mixed Glioma versus Oligodendroglioma

It is well recognized that a subset of gliomas demonstrate mixed features of oligodendroglioma and astrocytoma, so called oligoastrocytomas or mixed gliomas [2, 23] (Figures 17 and 18). The tumor patterns may be intermixed or the tumor may demonstrate geographic areas resembling one type or the other. Precise criteria for the diagnosis do not exist. People use parameters ranging from 20-35% of a second component to make the diagnosis. One can easily appreciate the challenge of assessing this in a tumor where the two components are admixed together. Rendering the diagnosis in small biopsies is also problematic, in that by doing so, one assumes that the biopsy is representative of the lesion as a whole. Gliomas are notoriously heterogenous lesions. It is not unusual to find small areas resembling astrocytoma in an oligodendroglioma and vice versa.

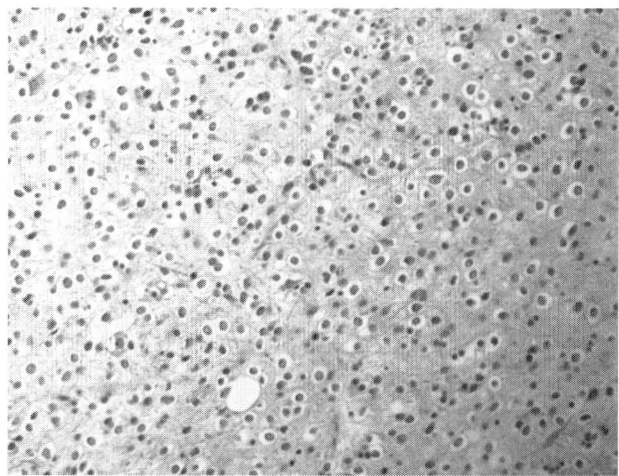

Figure 17. This tumor had areas resembling a low grade oligodendroglioma, WHO grade II (seen here) and other areas resembling a low grade diffuse astrocytoma (see Figure 18). The tumor was diagnosed as a low grade oligoastrocytoma (low grade mixed glioma) (hematoxylin and eosin, original magnification 200X).

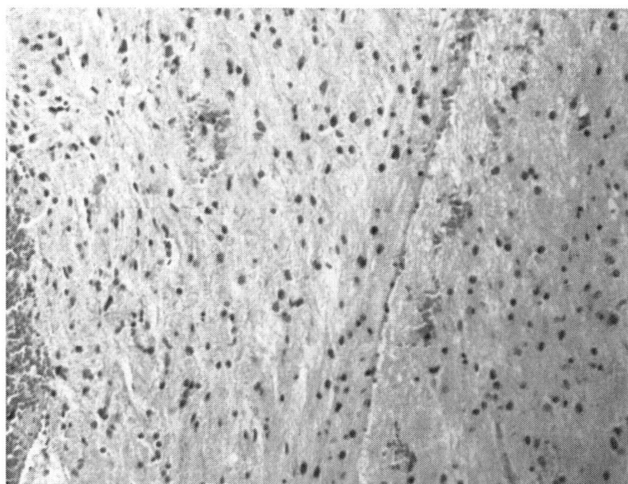

Figure 18. Another area of the same tumor as in Figure 17 showing a proliferation of cells with elongated, irregularly shaped nuclei, consistent with low grade astrocytoma (hematoxylin and eosin, original magnification 200X).

The designation is best employed in larger resection specimens. Oligoastrocytomas are graded as oligodendrogliomas are, as low grade (WHO grade II) and anaplastic (WHO grade III) lesions. The same histologic features which are used to grade astrocytomas and oligodendrogliomas are used to grade mixed tumors. In lesions with necrosis, a designation of glioblastoma with oligodendroglioma component is now favored (WHO grade IV).

This diagnosis is variably used in practice. In the last few years, given the increased information known about molecular genetics and brain tumors, there is a growing trend toward avoidance of the designation. Lesions which have the genetic signature of oligodendroglioma tend to behave like oligodendroglioma. Those that have the molecular profile of astrocytoma behave like astrocytoma. There is a sentiment among some that these tumors should be classified more along their molecular profile than their histologic phenotype.

PILOCYTIC ASTROCYTOMA VERSUS OLIGODENDROGLIOMA

Pilocytic astrocytomas represent a variant form of astrocytoma which has a unique clinical, molecular, and histologic phenotype [2, 24-25]. These tumors more frequently arise in younger age patients, where it is the most common glioma of childhood. They are often found to arise in certain locations including the cerebellum, brain stem, optic nerve and region around the thalamus and basal ganglia. On imaging, they typically are cystic with a mural nodule that enhances. Histologically, tumors may occasionally demonstrate areas that resemble oligodendroglioma with cells marked by rounded nuclei, scant cytoplasm and pericellular clearing (Figure 19). Most tumors, however, contain other areas in which the tumor cells are more elongated (piloid) in appearance. The tumor classically has a biphasic appearance with areas in which cells are more compactly arranged and other areas where the tumor has a looser, often microcystic appearance. The majority of tumors contain Rosenthal fibers (particularly in the more compact, fibrillary areas) which are tapered, corkscrew-shaped, eosinophilic structures (Figure 20). Many tumors also demonstrate eosinophilic granular bodies (especially in the looser areas) which are globular aggregates (Figure 21). Rosenthal fibers and granular bodies are not seen in oligodendrogliomas. Pilocytic astrocytomas generally demonstrate little or no mitotic activity, which correlates typically with low proliferation indices on Ki-67 immunostaining.

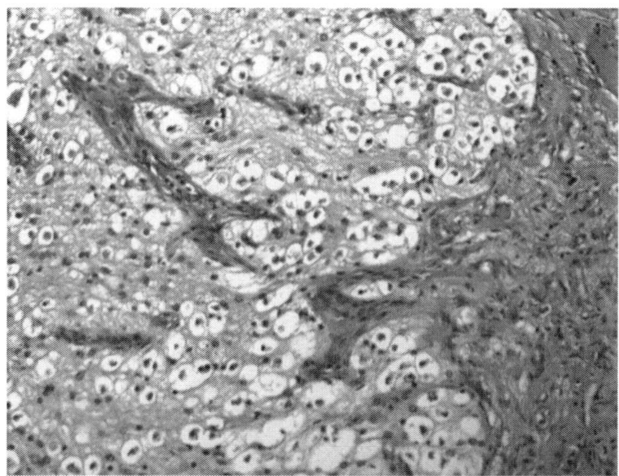

Figure 19. Some pilocytic astrocytomas, WHO grade I, may show areas marked by cells with more rounded nuclei, scant cytoplasm and pericellular clearing, resembling oligodendroglioma (hematoxylin and eosin, original magnification 200X).

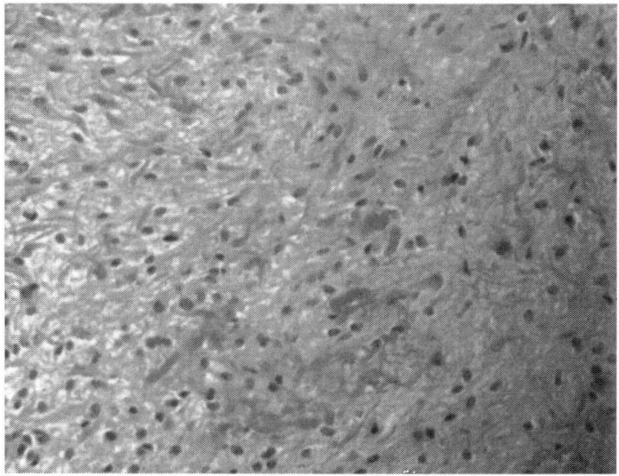

Figure 20. The majority (but not all) pilocytic astrocytomas demonstrate elongated, eosinophilic structures known as Rosenthal fibers; these are not a feature of oligodendrogliomas (hematoxylin and eosin, original magnification 400X).

They often contain areas of vascular proliferative change which accounts for the enhancement one sees on imaging in these tumors but the vascular changes are not associated with more aggressive behavior as it is in oligodendrogliomas. Nuclear pleomorphism may be focally quite pronounced in pilocytic astrocytomas, and that is acceptable. Necrosis is typically not a feature of pilocytic astrocytoma. Pilocytic astrocytomas do not demonstrate any of the molecular features of oligodendrogliomas such as chromosome 1p and 19q deletions and IDH-1 immunoreactivity. BRAF mutations are found in many pilocytic tumors [26-27].

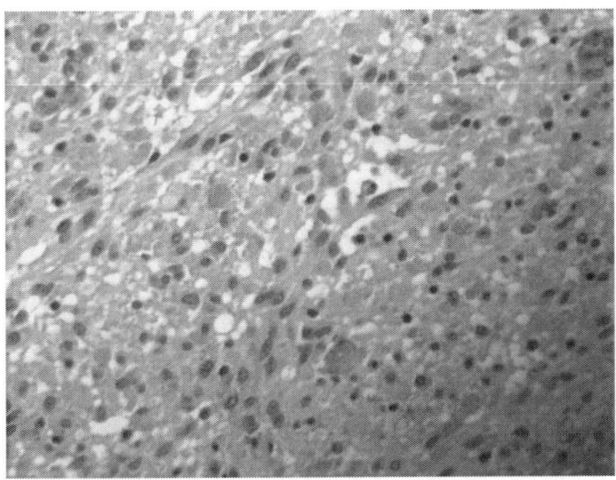

Figure 21. Similarly, a majority of pilocytic astrocytomas may also demonstrate eosinophilic granular bodies, a feature not seen in oligodendrogliomas (hematoxylin and eosin, original magnification 400X).

The importance in making the distinction lies in the differences in behavior and subsequently management. Pilocytic astrocytomas are considered WHO grade I lesions and are often amenable to surgical resection because they tend to be more circumscribed and less infiltrative than oligodendrogliomas. Adjuvant chemotherapy or radiation is not typically employed in treating most cases. There is a known association of pilocytic astrocytomas with Neurofibromatosis type I [28].

Papillary Glioneuronal Tumor versus Oligodendroglioma

The papillary glioneuronal tumor is a rare, relatively circumscribed lesion which generally behaves as a grade I neoplasm [29-31]. They arise in the cerebral hemispheres, most commonly in the temporal lobe. The tumor is marked by a prominent pseudopapillary architecture in which hyalinized vessels are surrounded by cuboidal glial cells (GFAP positive) (Figures 22 and

23). Intervening areas consist of collections of small rounded neurocytic cells, resembling oligodendrocytes. These neurocytic cells demonstrate strong positive staining with neural markers such as synaptophysin, neuron specific enolase, NeuN and class III beta-tubulin (Figure 24). These tumors do not demonstrate chromosome 1p deletions as seen in oligodendrogliomas.

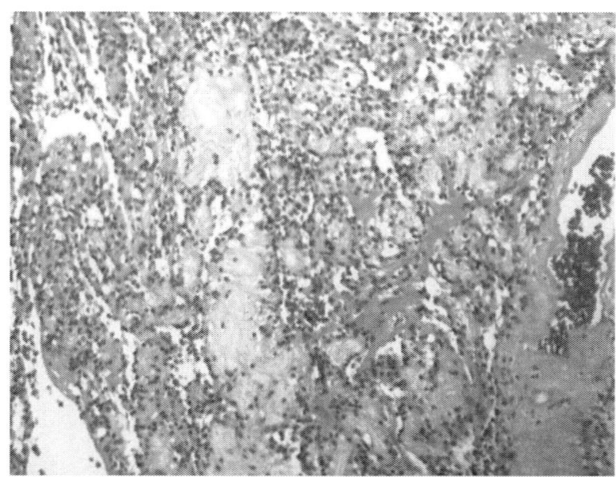

Figure 22. A rare tumor, the papillary glioneuronal tumor, is marked by blood vessels rimmed by GFAP positive glial cells, set against a background of rounded cells resembling oligodendrocytes which actually demonstrate neurocytic differentiation (synaptophysin positive) (hematoxylin and eosin, original magnification 200X).

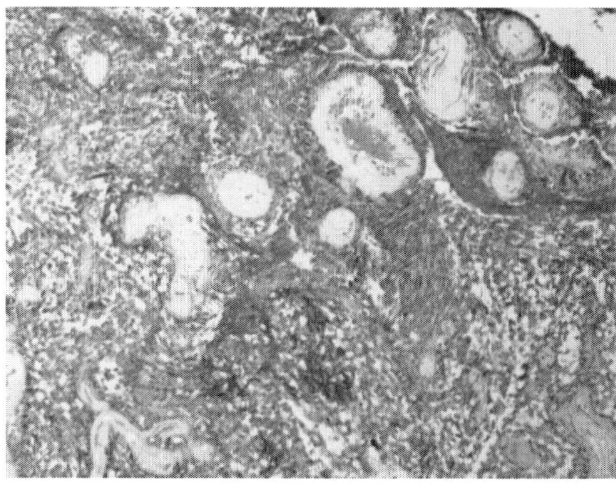

Figure 23. A papillary glioneuronal tumor stained with GFAP antibody and showing positivity in cells arranged around the blood vessels (GFAP, original magnification 200X).

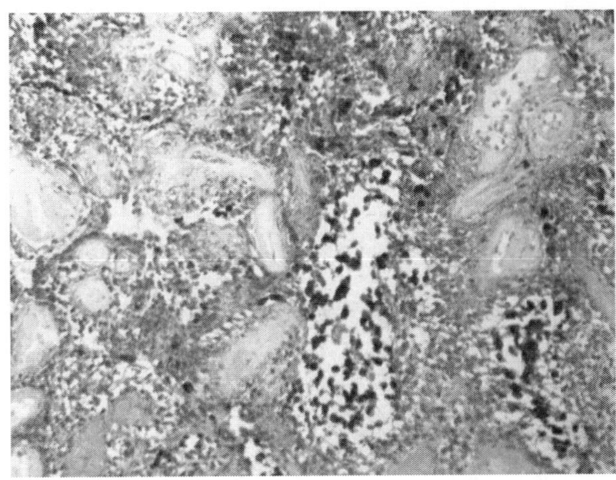

Figure 24. A papillary glioneuronal tumor stained with synaptophysin antibody demonstrating groups of neurocytic cells staining positively (synaptophysin, original magnification 200X).

DYSEMBRYOPLASTIC NEUROEPITHELIAL TUMOR VERSUS OLIGODENDROGLIOMA

The dysembryoplastic neuroepithelial tumor, or DNET for short, is a relatively uncommon, low grade glioneuronal neoplasm that morphologically can be impossible to distinguish from a microcystic low grade oligodendroglioma on a small biopsy. DNETs classically present in younger age patients with a history of pharmacoresistent epilepsy [32-36]. Although temporal lobe is the most common site of origin, the tumor has been described as arising throughout the cerebrum and in the cerebellum.

DNETs are typically circumscribed lesions, multinodular and cortical based (Figure25). The lesion often has a cystic/microcystic appearance and has been described as having the appearance of blistering on the surface the brain. The typical oligodendroglioma is a white matter based tumor that is uninodular and infiltrative. The primary cellular component of the DNET consists of rounded cells with scant cytoplasm resembling oligodendrocytes. These cells are admixed with normal appearing neuronal cells, hence the glioneuronal nature of these tumors. Cells are frequently arranged against a microcystic background. There is minimal atypia to either cellular component of the tumor.

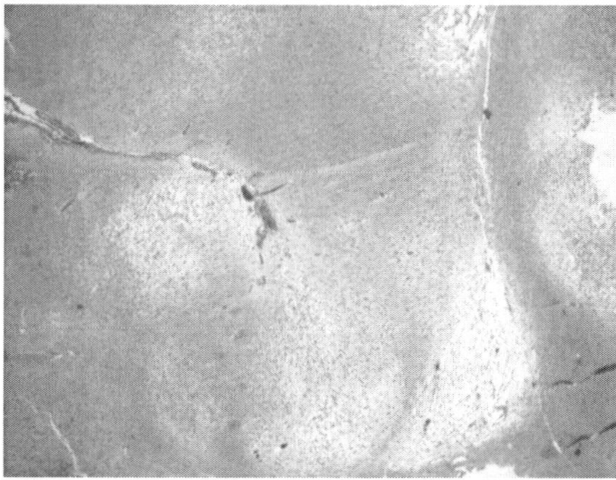

Figure 25. Low magnification appearance of a dysembryoplastic neuroepithelial tumor highlighting the tumor's typical multinodularity. Most of the tumor is cortical based (hematoxylin and eosin, original magnification 20X).

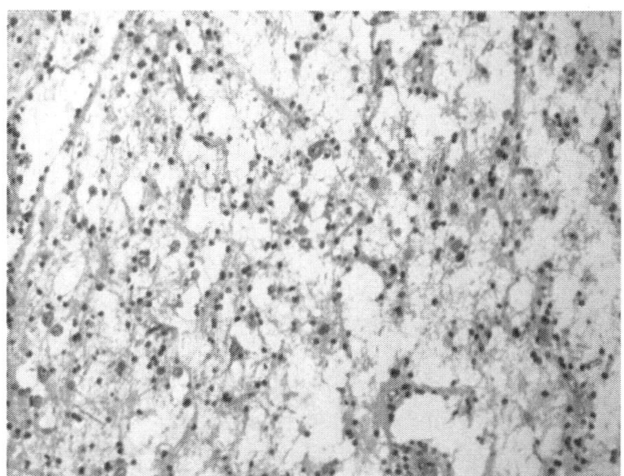

Figure 26. Dysembryoplastic neuroepithelial tumors consist of a proliferation of small rounded cells resembling oligodendrocytes with intermixed normal appearing neurons. Cells are typically arranged against a microcystic background (hematoxylin and eosin, original magnification 200X).

An arcuate capillary vascular pattern and occasionally microcalcifications may be encountered in DNETs, like in oligodendrogliomas. Occasional tumors may extend into the leptomeninges without any apparent impact on prognosis. (Figure 27). Most tumors, if one examines the cortical tissue next to them, demonstrate cortical architectural disorganization (focal cortical dysplasia).

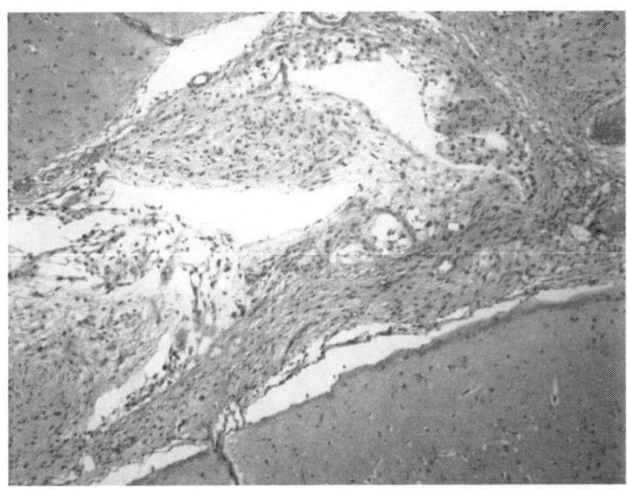

Figure 27. Occasional tumors extend to involve the leptomeninges; this does not appear to have an adverse prognosis (hematoxylin and eosin, original magnification 100X).

DNETs have an excellent prognosis and are amenable to surgical resection. They are designated as WHO grade I tumors. They demonstrate low rates of cell proliferation and low Ki-67 labeling indices. They lack IDH-1 immunoreactivity and lack deletions on chromosomes 1p and 19q [37].

From a practical perspective, in a small biopsy or fragmented specimen, it may be difficult or impossible to appreciate the multinodularity or cortical location of the lesion and confusion with oligodendroglioma is possible. It may not be possible to tell the two lesions apart, morphologically speaking. Use of molecular testing (chromosome 1p and 19q testing) or IDH-1 staining may be potentially helpful, especially if these tests are positive, which would favor oligodendroglioma. Negative test results are less informative.

Ganglioglioma versus Oligodendroglioma

Gangliogliomas, like DNETs, represent glioneuronal tumors and are most frequently encountered in the setting of medically intractable epilepsy arising in the temporal lobe [38-40]. Like DNETs, they generally represent WHO grade I lesions, which are fairly circumscribed and amenable to surgical excision.

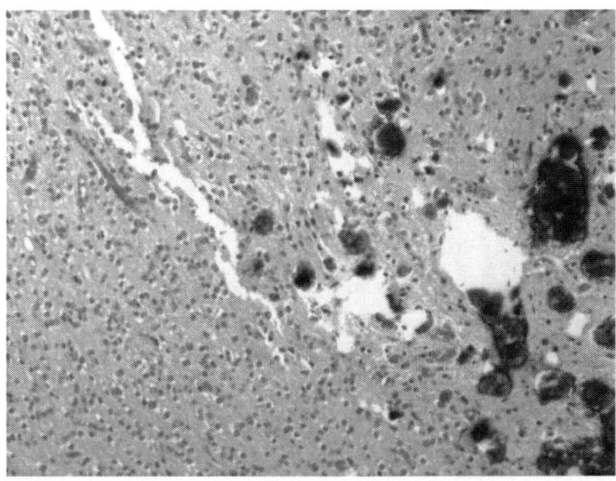

Figure 28. Gangliogliomas may contain focal areas, as seen here, in which the glioma component resembles an oligodendroglioma. Calcification is also present in this tumor (hematoxylin and eosin, original magnification 200X).

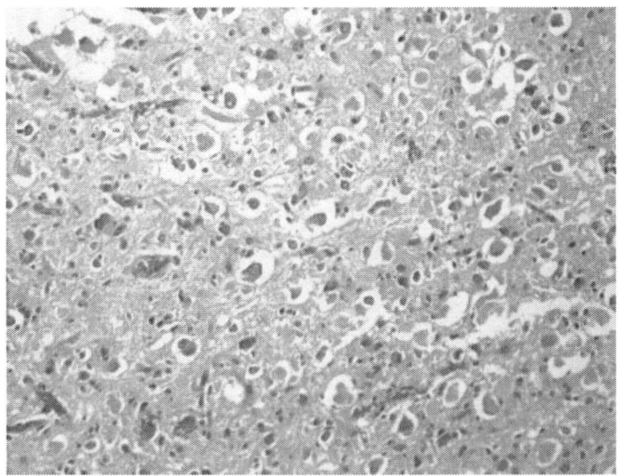

Figure 29. Gangliogliomas are marked by an atypical neuronal cell component which in some tumors may be only focally present (hematoxylin and eosin, original magnification 200X).

Histologically, gangliogliomas are marked by an admixture of a gliomatous component and an atypical neuronal cell or ganglion cell component. The glioma component most commonly resembles an astrocytoma. Occasional tumors may have gliomatous areas resembling a low grade oligodendroglioma (Figure 28). All tumors are marked by an accompanying atypical neuronal cell component which may manifest as an increased number of atypical neuronal cells, an abnormal configuration of cells and cytologically atypical neurons (Figure 29). The neuronal component may, at times, be only focally present in the tumor; this underscores the importance of extensive sampling of these tumors to ensure recognition of the neuronal cell component and to prevent an erroneous diagnosis of a grade II glioma. Other fairly frequently encountered histologic features of gangliogliomas include perivascular chronic lymphocytic inflammation, eosinophilic granular bodies, microcystic changes and microcalcifications. As is the case with DNETs, the cortical tissue adjacent to many gangliogliomas is marked by architectural disorganization (focal cortical dysplasia) (Figure 30), a feature not observed with oligodendrogliomas. Gangliogliomas lack the molecular features which are commonly observed in oligodendrogliomas.

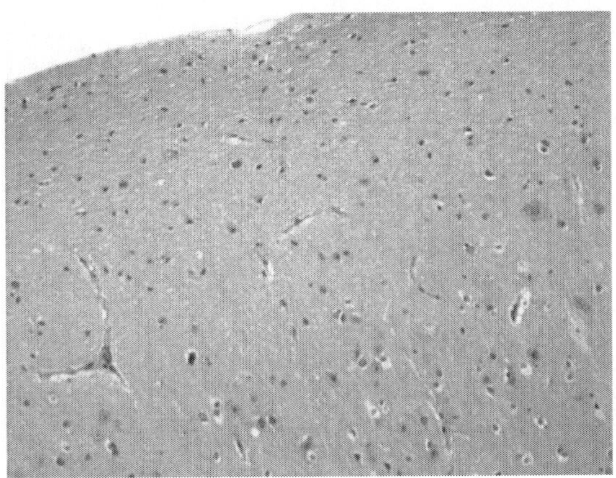

Figure 30. Many gangliogliomas are accompanied by adjacent cortical architectural abnormalities (focal cortical dysplasia). In this case, there was focal absence of cortical layer 2 and misplaced larger sized neurons high in the cortex (hematoxylin and eosin, original magnification 200X).

Central Neurocytoma versus Oligodendroglioma

Central neurocytomas are low grade lesions (WHO grade II) that typically present as an intraventricular masses, most commonly involving the lateral ventricles. Examples of extraventricular neurocytomas are well documented [42]. They are most commonly encountered in young adults and not surprisingly present with signs and symptoms related to increased intracranial pressure.

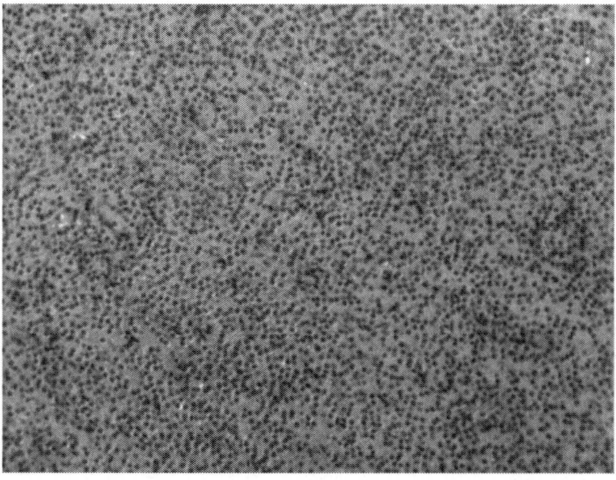

Figure 31. Central neurocytomas consist of sheets of rounded cells with scant cytoplasm, resembling oligodendroglioma (hematoxylin and eosin, original magnification 200X).

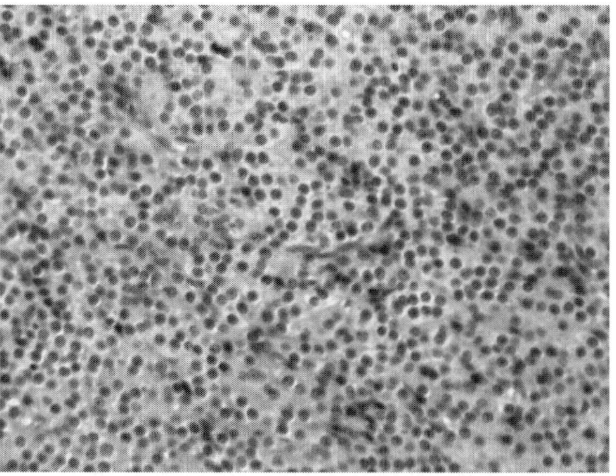

Figure 32. Nuclei in a central neurocytoma show a salt and pepper chromatin pattern, not typically seen in oligodendrogliomas (hematoxylin and eosin, original magnification 400X).

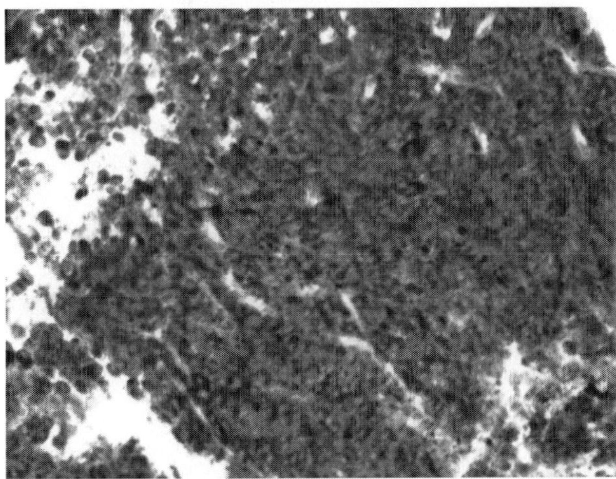

Figure 33. Central neurocytomas demonstrate diffuse positive staining with markers of neural differentiation such as seen here with synaptophysin (synaptophysin, original magnification 200X).

Histologically, tumors are marked by a proliferation of uniformly rounded cells with scant cytoplasm (Figure 21). Cell nuclei have a salt and pepper or finely speckled chromatin pattern and are typically devoid of large nucleoli (Figure 32). Capillary blood vessels, similar to oligodendroglioma, and microcalcifications may be present. Neurocytomas demonstrate diffuse immunoreactivity with markers of neural differentiation (Figure 33). Necrosis and vascular proliferative changes are typically absent. Low labeling indices, using cell proliferation markers, is common [43]. In rare cases, increased mitotic activity and vascular proliferative changes may be seen in so called atypical neurocytomas [44]; these lesions may be associated with a shorter recurrence free survival. These tumors again lack the genetic features commonly encountered in oligodendrogliomas.

Clear Cell Ependymoma versus Oligodendroglioma

Rare cases of ependymoma are marked by cells with rounded nuclei and perinuclear clearing, so called clear cell ependymoma [45-47] (Figure 34). This relatively uncommon variant preferentially arises in the supratentorial compartment of young patients. Sampling of these tumors sometimes uncovers areas demonstrating more classic true ependymal rosettes (tumor cells arranged around a space or lumen) or perivascular pseudorosettes (tumor cells arranged around a blood vessel) (Figures 35 and 36).

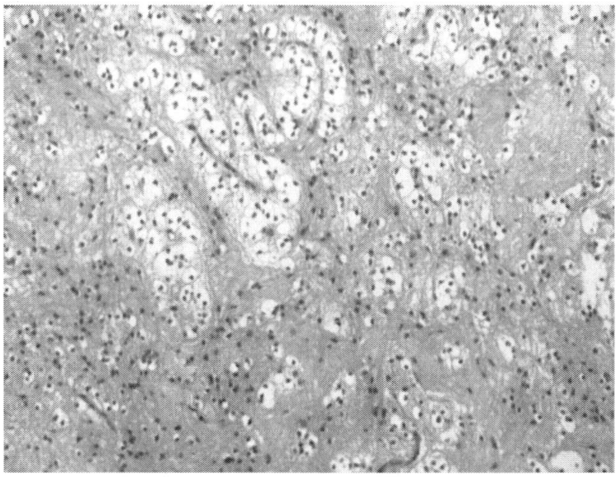

Figure 34. Rare ependymomas may contain areas such as this with rounded cells and pericellular clearing resembling oligodendroglioma (hematoxylin and eosin, original magnification 200X).

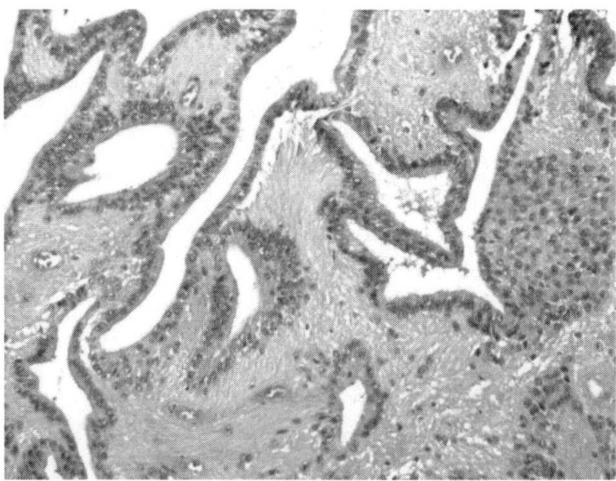

Figure 35. Typical ependymomas are characterized by the presence of true ependymal rosettes with ependymal cells arranged around spaces or channels, as seen here (hematoxylin and eosin, original magnification 200X).

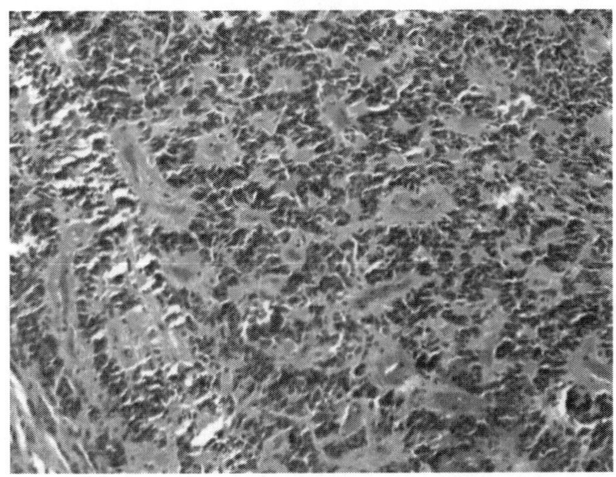

Figure 36. Ependymomas also frequently demonstrate perivascular pseudorosettes, as illustrated in this tumor (hematoxylin and eosin, original magnification 200X).

The intraventricular location of these tumors should be a tip off to a potential diagnosis. Immunoreactivity to epithelial membrane antigen (EMA) antibody is often present (not the case with oligodendrogliomas). Ultrastructurally, ependymomas are marked by cell junctions, microvilli and cilia with ciliary body attachments (blepharoplasts), none of which are present in oligodendrogliomas. Ependymal tumors, like oligodendrogliomas, are stratified into WHO grade II (low grade) and WHO grade III (anaplastic) tumors based on similar histologic parameters (increased mitotic activity, vascular proliferation and necrosis).

Rosette-forming Glioneuronal Tumor of the Fourth Ventricle versus Oligodendroglioma

The rosette-forming glioneuronal tumor of the fourth ventricle (RGNT) is a rare WHO grade I tumor which arises usually in adults in the midline, occupying the fourth ventricle or aqueduct [48-52]. Cases of similar appearing lesions arising elsewhere in the neuroaxis have been reported. These tumors are somewhat demarcated, although they may demonstrate focal areas of infiltration and are comprised of biphasic glial and neurocytic areas. The neural component, as we have seen in other neurocytic tumors, can resemble oligodendroglioma (Figure 37). The neurocytic component may contain neurocytic rosettes or perivascular pseudorosettes (Figure 38) and stain with neural antibodies.

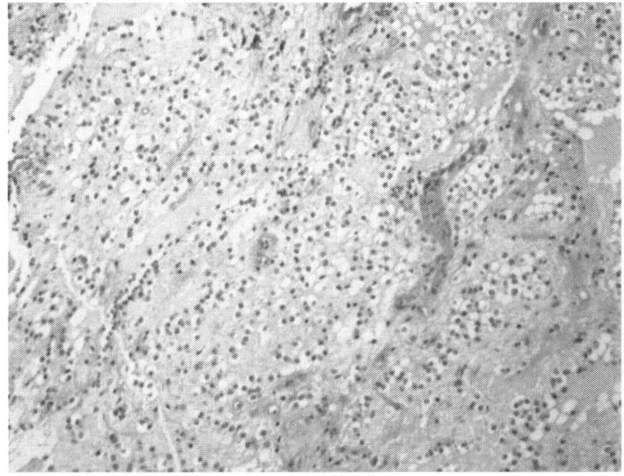

Figure 37. Rosette forming glioneuronal tumors of the fourth ventricle often resemble oligodendrogliomas (hematoxylin and eosin, original magnification 200X).

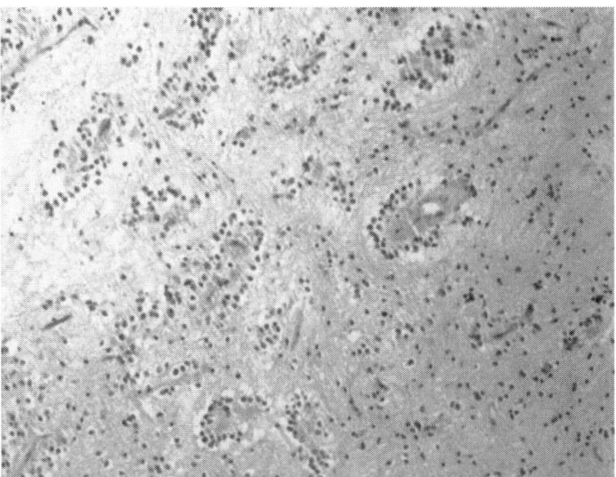

Figure 38. The presence of rosette structures, seen here, and the location of the tumor help differentiate this lesion from an oligodendroglioma (hematoxylin and eosin, original magnification 200X).

The glial component often predominates and most commonly resembles a pilocytic astrocytoma with stellate or spindled cells with elongated nuclei. In some tumors, the glial component may also resemble oligodendroglioma. Rosenthal fibers and eosinophilic granular bodies may be seen in these lesions. Low rates of cell proliferation and an absence of necrosis are typical. Vascular proliferative changes, similar to what one may encounter in pilocytic astrocytoma, may be seen in these tumors.

Inflammatory-Related Lesions versus Oligodendrogliomas

The last group of lesions that will be discussed in the histologic differential diagnosis of oligodendrogliomas includes lesions which contain inflammatory cells, particularly lymphocyte-rich lesions including lymphomas and macrophage-rich lesions such as demyelinating disease. Close attention to the histology usually results in a correct diagnosis. But when the histology may be confusing, immunohistochemistry using antibodies targeting lymphocytes (e.g., CD3 for T lymphocytes, CD20 for B lymphocytes or CD45 for both T and B lymphocytes) and macrophages (e.g., CD68) will easily resolve the confusion.

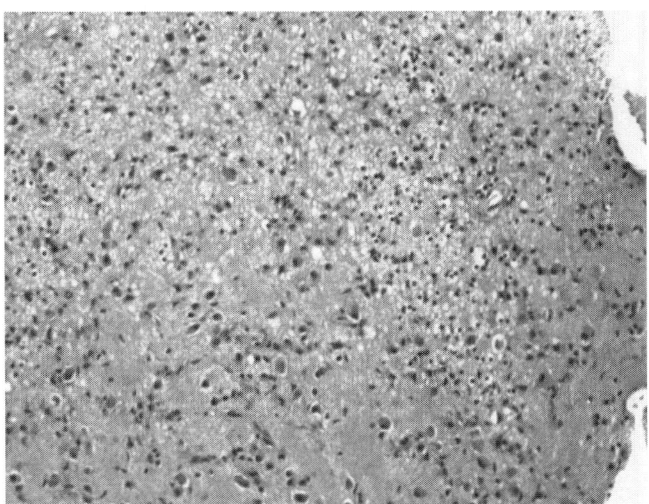

Figure 39. Small, benign appearing lymphocytes in an inflammatory condition such as encephalitis can show pericellular clearing (hematoxylin and eosin, original magnification 200X).

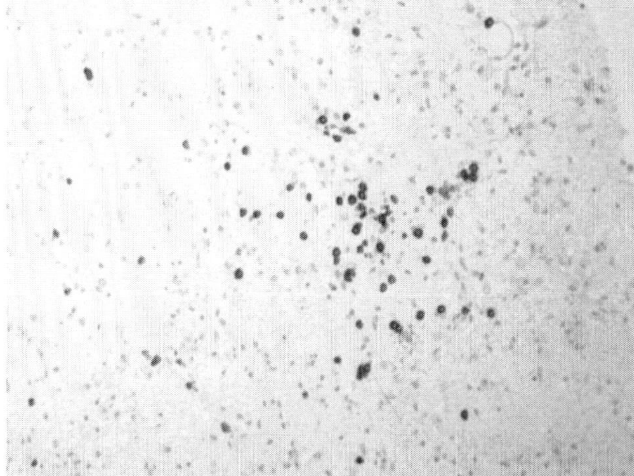

Figure 40. CD3 immunostain highlighting the T lymphocytes; oligodendrogliomas do not stain with lymphoid markers such as CD3. (original magnification 400X).

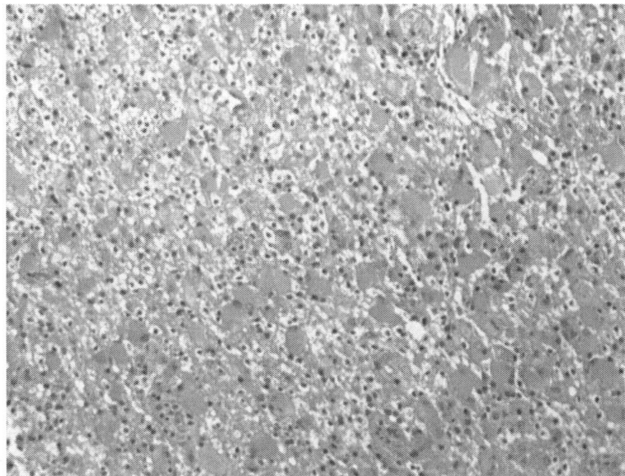

Figure 41. Macrophages in a demyelinating lesion, seen here, may ostensibly resemble an oligodendroglioma. Note the intermixed large eosinophilic reactive astrocytes (hematoxylin and eosin, original magnification 200X).

There are generally three scenarios which can give rise to confusion in this area. In the first, pericellular halos representing artifact may be seen around lymphocytes (Figures 39 and 40). Lymphocyte nuclei tend to be smaller and more hyperchromatic than oligodendroglial nuclei and they may be intermixed with other types of inflammatory cells which may be more easily recognizable.

They also tend to be seen in perivascular areas at all levels of the cerebrum (meninges, cortex as well as white matter).

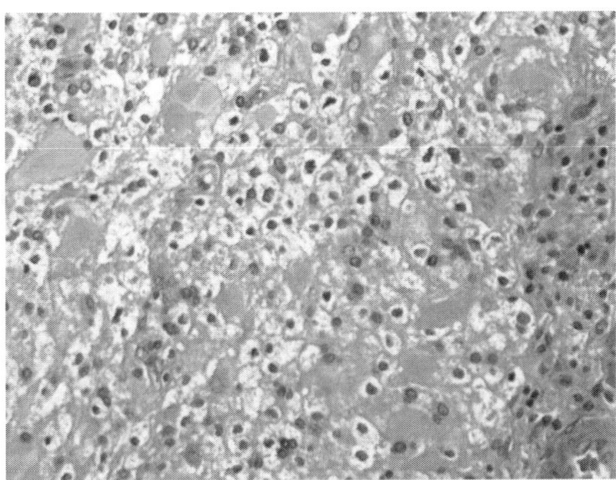

Figure 42. Close inspection of the cleared cells in a demyelinating lesion shows vacuolated cytoplasmic changes consistent with macrophages; immunostaining with macrophage directed antibodies such as CD68 can be helpful if needed (hematoxylin and eosin, original magnification 400X).

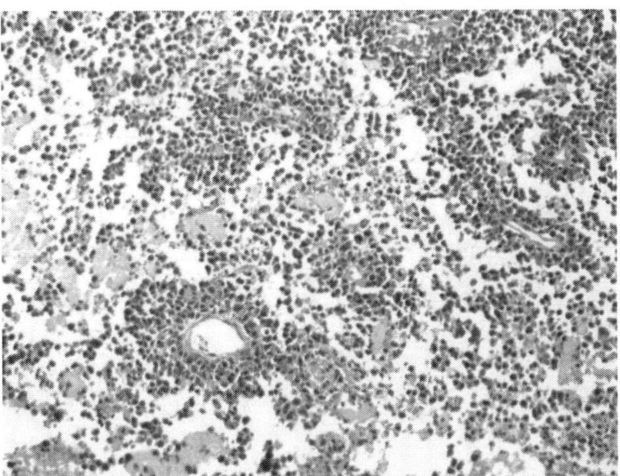

Figure 43. A non-Hodgkin's lymphoma, diffuse large B cell type, is seen here. The rounded but atypical appearing cells can be confused at times with an anaplastic oligodendroglioma. Immunostaining with CD20 antibody can be used to highlight the lymphoma cells (hematoxylin and eosin, original magnification 200).

In the second scenario, inflammatory cells at frozen section may be confused with glial cells. For example, macrophages in a demyelinating lesion at lower magnification may appear as cells with pericellular clearing, if one does not appreciate the vacuolated nature of the macrophage cytoplasm (Figures 41 and 42).

In the third scenario, primary central nervous system lymphoma may be confused with an anaplastic oligodendroglioma. Both tumor types may consist of sheets of atypical cells with a tendency to aggregate around blood vessels, have numerous mitotic counts and areas of necrosis (Figure 43). Most primary lymphomas in the brain represent diffuse large B cell lymphomas and will stain will immunomarkers such as CD20 [53].

CONCLUSION

There are a wide variety of central nervous system neoplasms and lesions that may have areas which morphologically resemble oligodendrogliomas. Careful attention to other histologic features in resected tumors and if needed, immunostaining or molecular testing can be employed and in most cases resolve the differential diagnosis. The importance of doing this lies in often significant differences in treatment approaches and outcomes.

REFERENCES

[1] Brat DJ. Overview of central nervous system anatomy and histology. In: *Neuropathology* (Prayson RA, ed.). Elsevier Saunders. Philadelphia, PA. 2012. pp. 1-39.

[2] Burger PC, Scheithauer BW. Tumors of the Central Nervous System. AFIP Atlas of Tumor Pathology Series 4. AFIP. Washington DC. 2007.

[3] Reifenberger G, Kros JM, Louis DN, et al. Oligodendroglioma and Anaplastic oligodendroglioma. In: WHO Classification of Tumours of the Central Nervous System (Louis DN, Ohgaki H, Weistler OD, Cavenee WK, editors). IARC Press. Lyons, FR. 2007. pp. 54-62.

[4] Dehghani F, Schachenmayr W, Laun A, et al. Prognostic implication of histopathological, immunohistochemical and clinical features of oligodendrogliomas: a study of 89 cases. *Acta Neuropathol.* 1998; 95: 493-504.

[5] Kros JM, Hop WC, Godschalk JJ, et al. Prognostic value of the proliferation-related antigen Ki-67 in oligodendrogliomas. *Cancer* 1994; 78: 1107-1113.

[6] Kros JM, Godschalk JJ, Krishnadath KK, et al. Expression of p53 in oligodendrogliomas. *J. Pathol.* 1993; 17: 285-290.

[7] Pavelic J, Hlavka V, Poljak M, et al. p53 immunoreactivity in oligodendrogliomas. *J. Neurooncol.* 1994: 22: 1-6.

[8] Nayak A, Ralte AM, Sharma MC, et al. p53 protein alterations in adult astrocytic tumors and oligodendroglioma. *Neurol. India* 2004; 52: 228-232.

[9] Capper D, Reuss D, Schittenhelm J, et al. Mutation-specific IDH1 antibody differentiates oligodendrogliomas and oligoastrocytomas from other brain tumors with oligodendroglioma-like morphology. *Acta Neuropathol.* 2011; 121: 241-252.

[10] Ichimura K, Pearson DM, Kocialkowski S, et al. IDH1 mutations are present in the majority of common adult gliomas but rare in primary glioblastomas. *Neuro-Oncology* 2009; 11: 341-347.

[11] Sahm F, Reuss D, Koelsche C, et al. Farewell to oligoastrocytoma: in situ molecular genetics favor classification as either oligodendroglioma or astrocytoma. *Acta Neuropathol.* 2014; 128: 551-559.

[12] Wiestler B, Capper D, Holland-Letz T, et al. ATRX loss refines the classification of anaplastic gliomas and identifies a subgroup of IDH mutant astrocytic tumors with better prognosis. *Acta Neuropathol.* 2013; 126: 443-451.

[13] Cairncross G, Jenkins R. Gliomas with 1p/19q codeletion: a.k.a. oligodendroglioma. *Cancer J.* 2008; 14: 352-357.

[14] Clark KH, Villano JL, Nikiforova MN, et al. 1p/19q testing has no significance in the workup of glioblastomas. *Neuropathol. Applied Neurobiol.* 2013; 39: 706-717.

[15] Kaneshiro D, Kobayashi T, Chao ST, et al. Chromosome 1p and 19q deletions in glioblastoma multiforme. *Appl. Immunohistochem. Mol. Morphol.* 2009; 17: 512-516.

[16] Brat DJ, Seiferheld WF, Perry A, et al. Analysis of 1p, 19q, 9p, and 10q as prognostic markers for high-grade astrocytomas using fluorescence in situ hybridization on tissue microarrays from Radiation Therapy Oncology Group trials. *Neuro. Oncol.* 2004; 6: 96-103.

[17] Perry A, Aldape KD, George DH, et al. Small cell astrocytoma: an aggressive variant that is clinicopathologically and genetically distinct from anaplastic oligodendroglioma. *Cancer* 2004; 101: 2318-2326.

[18] Nakamura M, Watanabe T, Yonekawa Y, et al. Promotor methylation of the DNA repair gene MGMT in astrocytomas is frequently associated with G:C – A:T mutations of the TP53 tumor suppressor gene. *Carcinogenesis* 2001; 22: 1715-1719.

[19] Ohgaki H. Genetic pathways to glioblastomas. *Neuropathology* 2005; 25: 1-7.

[20] Sadones J, Michotte A, Veld P, et al. MGMT promotor hypermethylation correlates with a survival benefit from temozolomide in patients with recurrent anaplastic astrocytoma but not glioblastoma. *Eur. J. Cancer* 2009; 45: 146-153.

[21] Prayson RA, Estes ML. Protoplasmic astrocytoma: A clinicopathologic study of 16 tumors. *Am. J. Clin. Pathol.* 1995; 103: 705-709.

[22] Prayson RA, Estes ML. MIB1 and p53 immunoreactivity in protoplasmic astrocytomas. *Pathol. Int.* 1996; 46: 862-866.

[23] Von Deimling A, Reifenberger G, Kros JM, et al. Oligoastrocytoma and Anaplastic oligoastrocytoma. In: WHO Classification of Tumours of the Central Nervous System (Louis DN, Ohgaki H, Weistler OD, Cavenee WK, editors). IARC Press. Lyons, FR. 2007. Pp. 63-67.

[24] Tihan T, Ersen A, Qaddoumi I, et al. Pathologic characteristic of pediatric intracranial pilocytic astrocytomas and their impact on outcome in 3 countries: a multi-institutional study. *Am. J. Surg. Pathol.* 2012; 36: 43-55.

[25] Collins VP, Jones DTW, Giannini C. Pilocytic astrocytoma: pathology, molecular mechanisms and markers. *Acta Neuropathol.* 2015; 129: 775-788.

[26] Berghoff AS, Preusser M. BRAF alterations in brain tumours: molecular pathology and therapeutic opportunities. *Curr. Opin. Neurol.* 2014; 27: 689-696.

[27] Schindler G, Capper D, Meyer J, et al. Analysis of BRAF V600E mutation in 1,320 nervous system tumors reveals high mutation frequencies in pleomorphic xanthoastrocytoma, ganglioglioma and extra-cerebellar pilocytic astrocytoma. *Acta Neuropathol.* 2011; 121: 397-405.

[28] Gutmann DH McLellan MD, Hussain I, et al. Somatic neurofibromatosis type I (NF1) inactivation characterizes NF1-associated pilocytic astrocytoma. *Genome Res.* 2013; 23: 431-491.

[29] Ishizawa T, Komori T, Shibahara J, et al. Papillary glioneuronal tumor with minigemistocytic components and increased proliferative activity. *Hum. Pathol.* 2006; 37: 627-630.

[30] Komori T, Scheithauer BW, Anthony DC, et al. Papillary glioneuronal tumor: a new variant of mixed neuronal-glial neoplasm. *Am. J. Surg. Pathol.* 1998; 22: 1171-1183.

[31] Tsukayama C, Arakawa Y. A papillary glioneuronal tumor arising in an elderly woman: a case report. *Brain Tumor Pathol.* 2002; 19: 35-39.

[32] Daumas-Duport C, Scheithauer BW, Chodkiewicz JP, et al. Dysembryoplastic neuroepithelial tumor: a surgically curable tumor of young patients with intractable partial seizures. Report of thirty-nine cases. *Neurosurgery* 1988; 23: 545-556.

[33] Pasquier B, Peoc'h M, Fabre-Bocquentin B, et al. Surgical pathology of drug resistant partial epilepsy: A 10-year experience with a series of 327 consecutive resections. *Epileptic Disord* 2002; 4: 99-119.

[34] Daumas-Duport C. Dysembryoplastic neuroepithelial tumours. *Brain Pathol.* 1993; 3: 283-295.

[35] Prayson RA, Estes ML. Dysembryoplastic neuroepithelial tumor. *Am. J. Clin. Pathol.* 1992; 97: 398-401.

[36] Prayson RA, Fong J, Najm I. Coexistent pathology in chronic epilepsy patients with neoplasms. *Mod. Pathol* 2010; 23: 1097-1103.

[37] Prayson RA, Castilla EA, Hartke M, et al. Chromosome 1p allelic loss by fluorescence in situ hybridization is not observed in dysembryoplastic neuroepithelial tumors. *Am. J. Clin. Pathol.* 2002; 118: 512-517.

[38] Luyken C, Blumcke I, Fimmers R, et al. The spectrum of long-term epilepsy-associated tumors: long-term seizure and tumor outcome and neurosurgical aspects. *Cancer* 2004; 101: 146-155.

[39] Prayson RA, Khajavi K, Comair YG. Cortical architectural abnormalities and MIB1 immunoreactivity in gangliogliomas: a study of 60 patients with intracranial tumors. *J. Neuropathol. Exp. Neurol.* 1995; 54: 513-520.

[40] Wolf HK, Muller MB, Spanle M, et al. Ganglioglioma: a detailed histological and immunohistochemical analysis of 61 cases. *Acta Neuropathol.* 1994; 88:166-173.

[41] Hassoun J, Soylemezoglu F, Gambarelli D, et al. Central neurocytoma: a synopsis of clinical and histological features. *Brain Pathol.* 1993; 3: 297-306.

[42] Giangaspero F, Cenacchi G, Losi L, et al. Extraventricular neoplasms with neurocytoma features: A clinicopathological study of 11 cases. *Am. J. Surg. Pathol.* 1997; 21: 206-212.

[43] Englund C, Alvord ED Jr., Folkerth RD, et al. NeuN expression correlates with reduced mitotic index of neoplastic cells in central neurocytomas. *Neuropathol. Appl. Neurobiol.* 2005; 31: 429-438.

[44] Von Deimling A, Janzier R, Kleihues P, et al. Patterns of differentiation in central neurocytoma: An immunohistochemical study of eleven biopsies. *Acta Neuropathol.* 1990; 79: 473-479.

[45] Fouladi M, Helton K, Dalton J, et al. Clear cell ependymoma: a clinicopathologic and radiographic analysis of 10 patients. *Cancer* 2003; 98: 2232-2244.

[46] Min KW, Scheithauer BW. Clear cell ependymoma: a mimic of oligodendroglioma: clinicopathologic and ultrastructural considerations. *Am. J. Surg. Pathol.* 1997; 21: 820-826.

[47] Kawano N, Yada K, Yagishita S. Clear cell ependymoma: A histological variant with diagnostic implications. *Virchows Archiv A. Pathol. Anat.* 1989; 415: 467-472.

[48] Jacques TS, Eldridge C, Patel A, et al. Mixed glioneuronal tumour of the fourth ventricle with prominent rosette formation. *Neuropathol. Appl. Neurobiol.* 2006; 32: 217-220.

[49] Komori T, Scheithauer BW, Hirose T. A rosette-forming glioneuronal tumor of the fourth ventricle: infratentorial form of dysembryoplastic neuroepithelial tumor? *Am. J. Surg. Pathol.* 2002; 26: 582-591.

[50] Preusser M, Diertrich W, Czech T, et al. Rosette-forming glioneuronal tumor of the fourth ventricle. *Acta Neuropathol.* 2003; 106: 506-508.

[51] Arai A, Sasayama T, Tamaki M, et al. Rosette-forming glioneuronal tumor of the fourth ventricle-case report. *Neurol. Med. Chir.* (Tokyo) 2010; 50: 224-228.

[52] Anan M, Inoue R, Ishii K, et al. A rosette-forming glioneuronal tumor of the spinal cord: the first case of a rosette-forming glioneuronal tumor originating from the spinal cord. *Hum. Pathol.* 2009; 46: 898-901.

[53] Deckert M, Paulus W. Malignant lymphomas. In: WHO Classification of Tumours of the Central Nervous System (Louis DN, Ohgaki H, Weistler OD, Cavenee WK, editors). IARC Press. Lyons, FR. 2007. pp. 188-192.

In: Oligodendrogliomas (ODs)
Editor: Chad Reeves

ISBN: 978-1-63484-278-5

Chapter 4

LESSONS LEARNED FROM AWAKE BRAIN FUNCTION MAPPING IN AGGRESSIVE MULTIMODAL RESECTION OF OLIGODENDROGLIOMAS

Joshua D. Burks[1], Andrew K. Conner[1], MD, Phillip A. Bonney[1], James D. Battiste[1], MD, Chad Glenn[1], MD, and Michael E. Sughrue[1,2,*], MD

[1]Department of Neurosurgery,
[2]Oklahoma Comprehensive Brain Tumor Clinic,
University of Oklahoma Health Sciences Center,
Oklahoma City, OK, US

ABSTRACT

Oligodendrogliomas are diffusely infiltrating tumors that grow through white matter pathways. While these tumors are deadly in the long term and should be treated operatively whenever possible, their predisposition for eloquent tracts requires a compromise between preserving function and resecting tumor. Modern techniques of investigating functional neuroanatomy have demonstrated the variability

[*] Corresponding Author: Michael E. Sughrue, Department of Neurological Surgery, University of Oklahoma Health Sciences Center, 1000 N Lincoln Blvd, Suite 4000, Oklahoma City, OK 73104, Tel: (405) 271-4912, Fax: (405) 271-3091, Email: michael-sughrue@ouhsc.edu.

of eloquent tracts, highlighting the misleading nature of Broca's and Wernicke's areas as fixed notions in modern neurosurgery. Given that traditional landmarks of functional neuroanatomy are too inconsistent to be used reliably in tumor patients, speech mapping is used intraoperatively to identify sites critical to language in order to preserve language function. The awake patient performs naming and other language functions with the help of a speech pathology team, while the surgeon conducts cortical and subcortical electric stimulation to map out and avoid eloquent brain areas. With this multidisciplinary care, the vast majority of patients are not harmed by surgery. Here we review speech mapping in oligodendroglioma operations and provide data regarding patient outcomes with these methods.

INTRODUCTION

Characterized by their slow growing and indolent, but eventually fatal, course, oligodendrogliomas (ODG) are clinically approached with goals vastly different from decades past. With improvements to surgical technique owing to better understanding of neural plasticity and functional neuroanatomy, patients now anticipate better outcomes. As our understanding of tumor genetics has improved, lending to improved chemotherapeutic effectiveness, so too have our methods for removing ODG with intra-operative mapping.

Most commonly a type of low-grade glioma (LGG), ODG consists of a heterogeneity grouping of tumor types both histologically and clinically [1]. LGG accounts for 15% of primary brain tumors in adults [2]. Among patients with LGG, those with ODG have been noted to live longer [3-5]. Reported incidence of ODG is 1.3 per 100,000 [6]. Most often presenting in patients with refractory seizures, ODGs can present with other vague symptoms like focal or cognitive deficits [6]. These tumors are readily identified by an increased signal intensity of T2-weighted magnetic resonance (MR) imaging without enhancement. Median survival from the time of diagnoses ranges between 3.5 and 11.3 years with surgery and chemotherapy, depending on tumor grade [7].

Once the diagnosis is made, a neurosurgeon is faced with a number of considerations to be addressed herein. In this review, we will examine speech mapping and the concept of neural plasticity within the context of a multi-disciplinary approach for treating ODG. We present our experiences in treating this disease and experiences described by others, and discuss the impact of these modalities on disease outcomes.

Role for Surgery

Extent of resection (EOR) has been shown to significantly correlate with overall survival (OS) in LGG [8-10], and numerous studies have suggested that maximum OS is attained with gross total resection (GTR) [8, 9]. Indeed, survival is directly correlated to EOR, which is most often described by a percentage of estimated overall tumor-mass removal. One series showed a 5-year OS of 97% following surgery with EOR greater than 90%, while surgery with EOR less than 90% had a 5-year survival of 76% [9]. Although no Level I evidence exists to support the role of EOR in slowing disease progression, best evidence in the form of multiple, large case series strongly supports that increasing EOR improves LGG patient survival [5, 8, 11].

Surgical intervention is of paramount importance because it improves progression-free survival (PFS) and delays malignant transformation. Surgical impact on PFS is greatest with a maximal EOR in patients with ODG, as EOR predicts PFS in patients with known pure ODG. Additionally, residual tumor volume is predictive of OS [11]. In one case series of patients with low-grade, insular gliomas an EOR ≥90% had a 5-year PFS of 88%, while an EOR <90% had a 5 year PFS of 69%. EOR has also been shown to predict malignant progression. In the same study, 5-year malignant progression free status was 88% for patients with ≥90% EOR, whereas it was 71% for those with an EOR <90% [8]. Surgery does not definitively change the biology associated with malignant transformation [11], but cytoreduction achieved in surgery ideally eliminates populations of cells that would otherwise progress to malignancy.

Oncofunctional Balance

While survival is best achieved with maximal EOR, clinicians must be cognizant of potential for loss of function with tumor removal. As areas of the brain important to language and motor functioning are often infiltrated by tumor in ODG, surgeons must navigate a tradeoff between quality of life and life prolongation. Few would argue for complete resection when a slight reduction in EOR could avoid leaving the patient severely disabled. Such considerations must preclude an over-zealous approach as ODGs have a predilection for functional areas. Approximately 83% of LGG are located within eloquent cortico-subcortical regions, with 27% involving the supplementary motor area and 25% invading the insula [12]. Additionally, 6% have been found in the primary somatosensory area and 4.5% involve the primary motor area [12].

Surgery carries important psychologic implications for patients. Patients undergoing surgery for primary brain tumors commonly experience affective mood disorders. Approximately 10% of all brain tumor patients are depressed pre-operatively, and 44% are depressed one year post-operatively [13]. Emotional factors have been shown to predict outcomes independent of tumor grade and surgical treatment. In fact, depressed LGG patients have a significantly shorter survival time than patients who are not depressed. One study found depressed LGG patients had a mean survival time of 3.3-5.8 years, compared to non-depressed LGG patients who had a mean survival time of 10.0-11.7 years [14]. Recognition and treatment of psychiatric comorbidities thus plays an important role in surgery patient outcomes.

Mapping

Oncofunctional balance is best achieved through intraoperative brain mapping. Intraoperative mapping has significantly reduced operative morbidity associated with brain tumor resection. Mapping is performed in patients with tumors in highly eloquent areas. Generally, the patient is either awake throughout or asleep at the beginning and end (and awake only while the surgeon is in vicinity of eloquent brain tissue). In our procedures, we keep patients awake for the duration of the resection to maximize safety and minimize the potent, confounding effects of anesthesia. However, the selected approach is usually dependent upon preferences of the surgeon and patient's ability to cooperate. In any case, the patient is awake for functional mapping of language and motor areas by direct electrical stimulation (DES). The patient performs language, motor, and cognitive tasks while direct contact with a bipolar probe creates an electric current in the area of interest. A site maps "positive" if any change is noted in the patient's ability to complete the tasks during stimulation of that cortex or subcortex.

Mapping has evolved since its initial implementation by neurosurgeons. Originally, it was used to treat refractory seizures, where the epileptic focus was identified intraoperatively through stimulation, then resected. Given the circumstances of its development, neurosurgeons historically performed DES mapping in tumor resection to identify areas essential for language function, which required a large cortical area of exposure and extensive mapping in an awake patient. In positive mapping, language sites in awake patients can be identified 95-100% of the time [15]. However, surgeons can work to remove tumor based on the absence of language and motor deficits with stimulation-induced motor and language function, often called "negative mapping." This allows for less exposure of brain tissue, shorter procedures, and less discomfort for the patient. Using this method, deficit-free rates higher than 98% have been achieved in patients undergoing LGG resection in highly eloquent areas [16]. The University of California at San Francisco group observed new language deficits in 1.6% of patients at 6 months post-operatively—even with new deficits occurring after surgery in 14.0% and worsened deficits in 8.4% in one week after surgery. Of these resections, 14% were grade II-III ODG [16].

In contrast, glioma resection without mapping has been shown to cause high rates of disability. Several retrospective studies have compared rates of language impairment in surgeries without functional mapping. Notably, severe language deficits were found in 17% of patients who underwent supratentoral LGG resection prior to routine intraoperative functional mapping [17]. Further, the quality of resection is much improved with mapping, as knowledge of functional boundaries permits a less-restricted surgical approach. In 100 patients undergoing resection for supratentoral LGG, 37% achieved subtotal resections and 6% were total. Yet in 122 patients at the same hospital undergoing resection with mapping, 50.8% were subtotal and 25.4% were total [17].

Anatomo-Functional Variability

Functional anatomy in patients presenting with glioma is often highly variable. This variability underscores the importance of mapping each individual undergoing tumor resection in an eloquent area. Especially in individuals with structural alterations secondary to gliomas, speech areas can vary greatly and are often not characterized by the traditional anatomic boundaries of Broca's area. In one major study that mapped speech in 186 patients, anomia sites were widely distributed throughout the frontal lobe, especially in the face-motor cortex. Additionally, few anomia sites were identified in the superior temporal gyrus also known as Wernicke's area [16]. Other studies have further shown the unreliability of Brodmann areas in understanding an individual's cortical functional anatomy [18-22].

PLASTICITY

Variability noted intraoperatively is best explained by the brain's plasticity. However, before examining plasticity, let us consider the framework that underlies our current understanding of neurophysiology. After all, early characterizations of neurophysiology created the foundation for a theory of neuroplasticity. Shortly before the turn of the century, D.O. Hebb proposed that learning and memory are based on the strengths of synapses between neurons, and that synaptic efficacy develops from repeated stimulation. This constitutes so-called "Hebbian theory." Which is to say: repeated stimulation alters baseline synaptic transmission, and consequently the activity of the downstream neuron. Researchers have built on Hebb's theory to propose three key mechanisms through which neurons produce effects [23]. These are summarized as: neuronal proliferation with branching; migration and differentiation; and organization through apoptosis and elimination of synapses [24]. Especially critical to the notion of plasticity is their coordinated proliferation and regulation; this is the notion that synapses not related to a stimulus are inhibited or eliminated by that stimulus [25]. One must also understand that neurons connected by a stimulus are coordinated temporally, meaning they fire synchronously in response to the same stimulus [26].

Repeated activation is responsible for structural, morphologic change. Support for morphologic change resulting from specific activation is documented in several well-known studies. Three-dimensional (3D) MR imaging in 26 pitch-perfect male orchestra players of the same handedness and IQ demonstrated significantly enlarged left inferior frontal gyrus (Broca's area) compared to controls, correcting for age. Additionally, researchers noted age-related volume reductions of grey matter in Broca's area and dorsolateral prefrontal cortex bilaterally in controls, but not in musicians [27]. Another study showed an enlarged hippocampus in taxi drivers compared to controls. Maguire and associates demonstrated that hippocampal volume correlated with time spent as a London taxi driver through structural MR imaging analysis [28]. As the hippocampus is believed to store spatial representation, its expansion in individuals with a high dependence on navigational skills is evidence further for plasticity in response to repeated stimuli.

Glial cells, long recognized as a key component of neuronal impulse timing, are also important in the neuronal regulation responsible for plasticity. Their subcortical modulatory effects on neuronal cell bodies and at synapses are necessary for plasticity. Astrocytes control the metabolism of neurons by controlling nutrient supply with varying levels of glutamate release [26].

Astrocytes control transmission at the synapse with glutamate as well [29]. Other glial cells are capable further of releasing neurotransmitters to communicate with one another and with neurons to form their own web of connectivity [30]. These inherent mechanisms of glial cells further explain the marked connectional reorganization of neurons in the presence of OGG and other LGGs.

In this framework, cortical plasticity is dependent upon sub-cortical, white-tract network interaction for reorganization following tumor resection [24]. A number of white-matter tracts have been elucidated as essential to language through subcortical mapping with direct electrostimulation (DES) intraoperatively with resection of LGG along said tracts. One mapping study of 115 patients found essential tracts include: 1) arcuate fasciculus, 2)inferior frontooccipital fasciculus, 3) subcallosal fasciculus, 4) frontoparietal phonological loop, and 5) fibers coming from the ventral premotor cortex [31]. Given that tumors were resected along these tracts with no safety margin, all 115 patients in the trail had speech deficits postoperatively. However, as the tracts remained intact, all but 2/115 patients in the study regained normal language by three months postoperatively [16]. Leaving the tracts intact allowed for reorganization of functional areas.

White-matter tract preservation is key to rehabilitative potential in patients following cortical injury, and white-tract conservation allows for a full recovery of function even after damage to eloquent cerebral cortex. That is to say, leaving subcortical structures intact allows for functional reorganization. Stroke studies first demonstrated that damage to language associated tracts results in more permanent aphasia than a corresponding cortical injury [32]. Since then, researchers have found redundancy of connections allows for short term plasticity, wherein neuronal synapses that were once silent in normal conditions become functional in pathologic states resulting from a lack of sensory input [24, 33]. And yet, functioning not immediately restored with short-term plasticity can be induced with repetitive stimuli in rehabilitation [34]. In a study by Liepert and associates, transcranial magnetic stimulation (TMS) imaging was performed on chronic stroke patients with stable right-sided paresis, and motor areas were mapped. Following therapy with constraint-induced movement (which restricts unaffected muscles to concentrate purposeful movements on the affected limb) of the right hand for 12 days, repeat imaging with TMS showed output shifts suggestive of recruitment of adjacent cortical areas to the area corresponding to hand-motor function. Imaging changes mirrored improved hand-motor performance [34].

Thus, reliance on new, intact subcortical pathways is inducible by repetitive exercises, resulting in cortical reorganization.

SELECTED CASES

Intriguing cases demonstrative of plasticity secondary to development of OGD are well documented in the literature. Plasticity is often best appreciated in the distorted anatomy in patients with slow-growing LGG. The cerebrum has more time to rearrange in these patients—as opposed to cerebral infarction wherein functional tissue loss is rapid in onset. Hayashi and colleagues describe a 36-year-old right handed patient with a WHO grade II ODG located in the right primary motor cortex, detected on MRI and confirmed by open biopsy. Awake surgery was performed with DES mapping and monitoring of somatosensory-evoked potentials (SEPs). SEPs are measured by recording electric current through the scalp while applying electrical stimulation to the skin over peripheral nerves of the upper extremity, and are an accurate, non-invasive way to detect primary somatosensory cortex [35]. The primary somatosensory area was identified in this manner, and the functional motor area mapped with DES [36]. The ODG was removed under continuous direct cortical and subcortical stimulations until positive mapping occurred, revealing that the motor function site had moved posteriorly across the central sulcus. Half of the tumor was not resected to preserve motor function as demonstrated with mapping. No motor deficit was noted post-operatively, and the patient remained seizure free, returning to his prior level of professional functioning [36].

In our own experience, brain plasticity plays a key role in our approach to treating patients with ODG. Functional reorganization of the primary motor cortex in patients with a long history of LGG is commonly encountered. In one such case, a 48-year-old right-handed woman presented with recurrence of ODG of the posterior left frontal lobe. The original tumor is shown in figure 1a. One year after the first operation, MRI showed a hyperintense T2 signal extending into the left lateral precentral gyrus and subcortical white matter of the precentral gyrus, postcentral gyrus, subcentrallobule, and supramarginal gyrus. Awake surgery and mapping were performed, followed by corticectomy on the tumor. Resection was performed until speech and motor tracts were encountered, achieving an EOR of 98-100%. We removed the primary motor cortex on the left side as can be seen in Figure 1b, and at discharge she was moving all extremities and had only a mild right facial weakness.

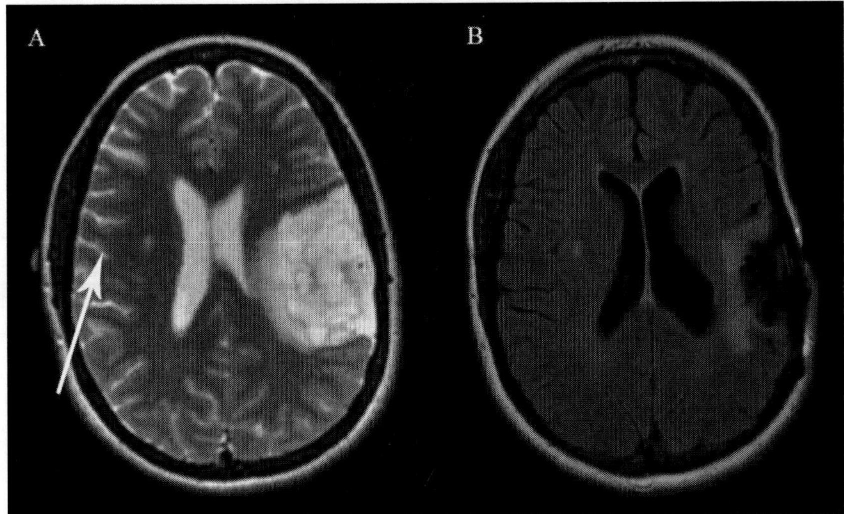

Figure 1. a: Pre-operative T2-weighted MR image showing large tumor mass involving the left lateral precentral gyrus and subcortical white matter of the precentral gyrus and postcentral gyrus lobe. The central sulcus is indicated on the right by an arrow. b: Post-operative T1-weighted MR image with contrast following awake surgery and mapping. Note the absence of the precentral gyrus on the left. The patient's only neurologic deficit at discharge was mild right facial weakness.

In light of the brain's plastic potential, patients can also benefit from a multi-step approach to tumor resection. Robles and colleagues have previously proposed moving beyond the traditional practice of one surgery for tumors in eloquent areas in favor of utilizing the natural course of gliomas to optimize therapy and quality of life [37]. They describe a 38-year-old right-handed woman presenting with refractory seizures secondary to grade II ODG in the left middle frontal gyrus (dorsal premotor cortex). Functional magnetic resonance imaging (fMRI) demonstrated language activation in the left frontal lobe, very close to the tumor with moderate recruitment of the right hemisphere in the lateral frontal cortex. The first surgery was performed preserving areas where DES resulted in speech arrest. Five years later, a second surgery on the same patient confirmed that functional centers had shifted slightly posteriorly, allowing for resection of the anterior part of the prefrontal gyrus. Luckily, biopsy at that time again showed grade II ODG, confirming the tumor had not undergone malignant transformation. Speech remained intact postoperatively, and at one-year follow-up examination no tumor recurrence was observed.

A second patient described by Robles had a grade II ODG likewise involving the left middle frontal gyrus [37]. In that case, the tumor was demonstrated to contain tissue associated with language functioning. The tumor was removed sparing the primary motor area, inferior frontal gyrus, and ventral premotor area to preserve functionality. Four years later, fMRI was performed, demonstrating a predominance of left-sided language function, which was similar to imaging performed before the first surgery. However, lateral frontal language functioning had shifted to the right hemisphere, again suggesting reorganization with tumor progression. Unlike the first operation, during the second operation, DES showed no response in the posterior part of the tumor, allowing for an additional 6cm^3 resection. Biopsy at that time demonstrated no evidence of malignant progression, and at one year post-operatively the patient had resumed normal professional activity.

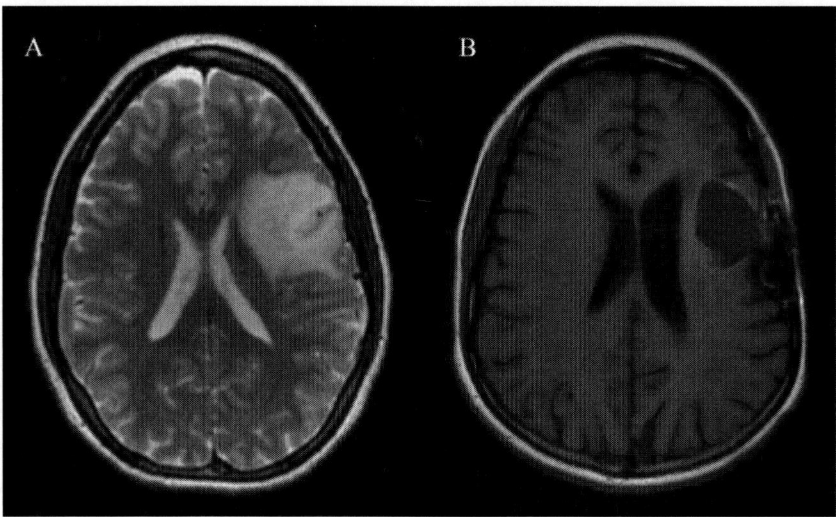

Figure 2. a: Pre-operative T2-weighted MR image showing tumor extending into the left inferior gyrus (Broca's area) and middle frontal gyrus, and along the margin of the external capsule. b: T1-weighted MR image with contrast after re-operation and resection of the tumor from the left inferior gyrus to the center of the middle frontal gyrus and the edge of the pre-central gyrus. The area that mapped positive for speech in a prior operation was no longer eloquent and allowed for complete resection with no postoperative speech deficits.

Here we report a similar case where we operated twice on a 24-year-old right-handed woman with ODG occupying speech areas on the left side. In this patient, a delayed second surgery allowed for complete removal of tumor even with infiltration of highly eloquent regions. She presented with seizures and concurrent postictal language difficulties, and was found on imaging to have tumor extending into the left inferior (Broca's area) and middle frontal gyri and along the margin of the external capsule as shown in Figure 2a. We performed awake surgery to resect the tumor, which included Broca's area. Resection was stopped after 90-95% of the tumor was removed when language centers were encountered. Speech arrest occurred with stimulation on the posterior side of the tumor, and facial motor function with stimulation on the medial edge of the tumor. The patient had no postoperative speech deficits. When surgery was repeated nine months later for re-growth, the area that mapped positive for speech during the last procedure was no longer eloquent. This allowed for tumor resection to the edge of the pre-central gyrus and up to the center of the middle frontal gyrus to obtain a complete resection. Post-operative imaging is shown in figure 2b.

ALTERNATIVES TO INTRA-OPERATIVE MAPPING

The role for awake surgery with intraoperative mapping in treating patients with ODG is further underscored by the mapping limitations of currently available non-invasive approaches. Current imaging modalities are not reliable enough in reproducing white-tract anatomy or in mapping functional anatomy to replace intraoperative mapping with DES. Diffusion tensor imaging and fiber tractography (DTI-FT) are MR imaging modalities that work through measuring water diffusion in myelinated fibers. DTI-FT provide three-dimensional reconstructions of white-matter tracts and can be used in preoperative planning for OGD resection. But the use of DTI-FT for intraoperative guidance has not been validated, owing to its technical limitations. The first is an inability of the study to resolve white-matter tract directionality in areas where multiple fiber bundles occupy the same voxel, or point in space [38]. Unfortunately, this type of architecture is common within an infiltrative tumor such as ODG. DTI-FT also requires identification of regions of interest based on normal anatomical locations, which may be altered in the presence of a tumor—leading to inaccurate mapping. Use of DTI-FT also requires consideration of brain shift intraoperatively as tumor mass is removed. Accuracy can be improved with intraoperative MR imaging (ioMRI), but this is both time consuming and expensive [38].

Despite its limited use intraoperatively, DTI-FT used in conjunction with mapping has been shown to reduce duration of mapping and the number of intraoperative seizures. A series of awake resections of LGG and HGG in 64 patients found that DTI-FT use in operative planning reduced the duration of resection (excluding craniotomy and closure) from 1 hour and 40 minutes to 1 hour and 3 minutes when subcortical motor mapping was performed. When language and motor DTI-FT mapping was applied, surgical duration was reduced from 2 hours and 30 minutes to 1 hour and 10 minutes. Additionally, intraoperative electrical and clinical seizure rates were significantly reduced [38].

Studies correlating fMRI data with direct brain mapping also have not proven useful in surgical planning. With respect to language, fMRI cannot be used in surgical decision making in the absence of intraoperative mapping. Functional MRI has demonstrated a poor sensitivity for detecting centers essential to naming and verb generation (66%) [39]. Most notably, naming demonstrates poor localization on fMRI in both frontal and temporoparietal areas [39]. One group has noted that fMRI sensitivity for speech centers can be increased with more activation tasks: word reading, visual and auditory verb generation, and listening to single words and text. This study, however, maintains a poor specificity for language centers[40].

SURGICAL ADJUVANTS

Research in the last decade has yielded techniques for definitive diagnosis and treatment based on immunohistochemistry. Histologic determination is important because it guides chemotherapeutic decisions. The World Health Organization provides a structure for histologically describing ODG. Based on classification by the WHO, grade II oligodendroglioma is categorized as LGG, which also includes grades I-II astrocytoma, and mixed oligoastrocytoma. Oligodendroglioma can also be grade III, referred to as high-grade, or anaplastic oligodendroglioma [1]. AO follows a more aggressive course, but is responsive to chemotherapy and radiation [6]. The WHO controversially recognizes a separate category for glioblastoma with features of ODG. Some pathologists recognize these tumors as a grade IV oligodendroglioma where others endorse a subset of glioblastoma [41]. Furthermore, astrocytoma tumors of all grades have been noted to contain oligodendroglial cells [11].

Combined with histologic categorization, better genetic characterization of ODG has heralded improved, targeted medical therapy. Patients with ODG have the greatest overall survival with surgical tumor resection and targeted chemotherapy [41]. Two landmark clinical trials have established a standard of care regimen for patients with newly diagnosed OGD. One found an OS of 42.3 months in patients with newly diagnosed OGD treated with procarbazine, lomustine, and vincristine (PCV) and radiotherapy (RT), compared to an OS of 30.6 in those treated with RT alone [7]. Patients without 1p/19q co-deletion have a poorer prognosis and follow a course more similar to oligoastrocytoma and pure astrocytoma tumors. A major predictor of response is 1p/19q allelic loss of anaplastic oligodendroglioma to combination radiation and chemotherapy at the time of diagnosis. Specifically, pure oligodendroglioma tumor patients with the 1p/19q are shown to benefit more from therapy with PCV [6]. Survival in patients with co-deleted OGD is 121 months, while those without 1/19q have an average survival of 101 months [42]. Mean survival is 84 months with the deletion and 33.6 months without when components of AO and AOA are present [43].

Additional tumor characteristics are important to the progression and prognosis of ODG. Oligodendrogliomas lacking deletion tend to instead have deletion of 9q21.3 (CDKN2A) and amplification of EGFR, CDK4, and other genes common to astrocytomas [44]. IDH mutations also correlate with poorer outcomes [7]. Angiogenesis has also been identified as a particularly useful prognostic value and indicates a need for more aggressive therapy. The presence of VEGF is predictive of poorer prognosis in any grade of oligodendroglioma [45]. Four more independent poor prognostic factors have been identified. These are: necrosis, absence of seizure, increased vascularization, and age >55 years [24, 46]. Assessing 1p/19q status in conjunction with histologic and radiologic markers of angiogenesis thus enables specific therapy for each oligodendroglioma tumor with a reasonable expectation for therapeutic response. Surgery, in conjunction with testing for these markers of progression, allows for targeted therapy that maximizes potential for favorable outcomes.

Conclusion

Taken together, our present understanding of ODG biology, cerebral plasticity and utilization of awake surgical mapping allow us to offer clear therapeutic benefit to patients—individuals for whom the best treatment path was murky at best just a decade ago. We believe the cases and findings presented in this review outline a clear way forward in the management of this disease, and emphasize the potential for ever-improving prognoses in patients diagnosed with ODG.

REFERENCES

[1] Thurnher MM. 2007 World Health Organization classification of tumours of the central nervous system. *Cancer Imaging*. 2009;9 Spec No A:S1-3.

[2] Ostrom QT, Gittleman H, Liao P, Rouse C, Chen Y, Dowling J, et al. CBTRUS statistical report: primary brain and central nervous system tumors diagnosed in the United States in 2007-2011. *Neuro. Oncol.* 2014;16 Suppl 4:iv1-63.

[3] Jaeckle KA. Oligodendroglial tumors. *Semin Oncol*. 2014;41(4):468-77.

[4] Sanai N, Chang S, Berger MS. Low-grade gliomas in adults. *J. Neurosurg*. 2011;115(5):948-65.

[5] Ahmadi R, Dictus C, Hartmann C, Zurn O, Edler L, Hartmann M, et al. Long-term outcome and survival of surgically treated supratentorial low-grade glioma in adult patients. *Acta Neurochir (Wien)*. 2009; 151(11):1359-65.

[6] Van den Bent MJ, Reni M, Gatta G, Vecht C. Oligodendroglioma. *Crit Rev. Oncol. Hematol*. 2008;66(3):262-72.

[7] Ohgaki H, Kleihues P. Population-based studies on incidence, survival rates, and genetic alterations in astrocytic and oligodendroglial gliomas. *J. Neuropathol. Exp. Neurol*. 2005;64(6):479-89.

[8] Sanai N, Polley MY, Berger MS. Insular glioma resection: assessment of patient morbidity, survival, and tumor progression. *J. Neurosurg*. 2010;112(1):1-9.

[9] Smith JS, Chang EF, Lamborn KR, Chang SM, Prados MD, Cha S, et al. Role of extent of resection in the long-term outcome of low-grade hemispheric gliomas. *J. Clin. Oncol*. 2008;26(8):1338-45.

[10] Chaichana KL, McGirt MJ, Laterra J, Olivi A, Quinones-Hinojosa A. Recurrence and malignant degeneration after resection of adult hemispheric low-grade gliomas. *J. Neurosurg*. 2010;112(1):10-7.

[11] Snyder LA, Wolf AB, Oppenlander ME, Bina R, Wilson JR, Ashby L, et al. The impact of extent of resection on malignant transformation of pure oligodendrogliomas. *J. Neurosurg*. 2014;120(2):309-14.

[12] Duffau H, Capelle L. Preferential brain locations of low-grade gliomas. *Cancer*. 2004;100(12):2622-6.

[13] D'Angelo C, Mirijello A, Leggio L, Ferrulli A, Carotenuto V, Icolaro N, et al. State and trait anxiety and depression in patients with primary brain tumors before and after surgery: 1-year longitudinal study. *J. Neurosurg*. 2008;108(2):281-6.

[14] Mainio A, Tuunanen S, Hakko H, Niemela A, Koivukangas J, Rasanen P. Decreased quality of life and depression as predictors for shorter survival among patients with low-grade gliomas: a follow-up from 1990 to 2003. *Eur Arch. Psychiatry Clin. Neurosci.* 2006;256(8):516-21.

[15] Ojemann G, Ojemann J, Lettich E, Berger M. Cortical language localization in left, dominant hemisphere. An electrical stimulation mapping investigation in 117 patients. 1989. *J. Neurosurg.* 2008;108(2):411-21.

[16] Sanai N, Mirzadeh Z, Berger MS. Functional outcome after language mapping for glioma resection. *N. Engl. J. Med.* 2008;358(1):18-27.

[17] Duffau H, Lopes M, Arthuis F, Bitar A, Sichez JP, Van Effenterre R, et al. Contribution of intraoperative electrical stimulations in surgery of low grade gliomas: a comparative study between two series without (1985-96) and with (1996-2003) functional mapping in the same institution. *J. Neurol. Neurosurg. Psychiatry.* 2005;76(6):845-51.

[18] Caspers S, Geyer S, Schleicher A, Mohlberg H, Amunts K, Zilles K. The human inferior parietal cortex: cytoarchitectonic parcellation and interindividual variability. *Neuroimage.* 2006;33(2):430-48.

[19] Rajkowska G, Goldman-Rakic PS. Cytoarchitectonic definition of prefrontal areas in the normal human cortex: II. Variability in locations of areas 9 and 46 and relationship to the Talairach Coordinate System. *Cereb. Cortex.* 1995;5(4):323-37.

[20] Tyler LK, Marslen-Wilson WD, Randall B, Wright P, Devereux BJ, Zhuang J, et al. Left inferior frontal cortex and syntax: function, structure and behaviour in patients with left hemisphere damage. *Brain.* 2011;134(Pt 2):415-31.

[21] Tymofiyeva O, Ziv E, Barkovich AJ, Hess CP, Xu D. Brain without anatomy: construction and comparison of fully network-driven structural MRI connectomes. *PLoS One.* 2014;9(5):e96196.

[22] Uylings HB, Rajkowska G, Sanz-Arigita E, Amunts K, Zilles K. Consequences of large interindividual variability for human brain atlases: converging macroscopical imaging and microscopical neuroanatomy. *Anat. Embryol. (Berl).* 2005;210(5-6):423-31.

[23] Hebb DO. *The Organization of Behavior.* New York, NY: Wiley; 1948.

[24] Saito A, Nakazato Y. Evaluation of malignant features in oligodendroglial tumors. *Clin. Neuropathol.* 1999;18(2):61-73.

[25] Favero M, Cangiano A, Busetto G. Hebb-based rules of neural plasticity: are they ubiquitously important for the refinement of synaptic connections in development? *Neuroscientist.* 2014;20(1):8-14.

[26] Bonvento G, Sibson N, Pellerin L. Does glutamate image your thoughts? *Trends Neurosci*. 2002;25(7):359-64.

[27] Sluming V, Barrick T, Howard M, Cezayirli E, Mayes A, Roberts N. Voxel-based morphometry reveals increased gray matter density in Broca's area in male symphony orchestra musicians. *Neuroimage*. 2002;17(3):1613-22.

[28] Maguire EA, Gadian DG, Johnsrude IS, Good CD, Ashburner J, Frackowiak RS, et al. Navigation-related structural change in the hippocampi of taxi drivers. *Proc. Natl. Acad. Sci. USA*. 2000;97(8):4398-403.

[29] Araque A, Parpura V, Sanzgiri RP, Haydon PG. Glutamate-dependent astrocyte modulation of synaptic transmission between cultured hippocampal neurons. *Eur. J. Neurosci*. 1998;10(6):2129-42.

[30] Haydon PG. GLIA: listening and talking to the synapse. *Nat. Rev. Neurosci*. 2001;2(3):185-93.

[31] Duffau H, Peggy Gatignol ST, Mandonnet E, Capelle L, Taillandier L. Intraoperative subcortical stimulation mapping of language pathways in a consecutive series of 115 patients with Grade II glioma in the left dominant hemisphere. *J. Neurosurg*. 2008;109(3):461-71.

[32] Naeser MA, Palumbo CL, Helm-Estabrooks N, Stiassny-Eder D, Albert ML. Severe nonfluency in aphasia. Role of the medial subcallosal fasciculus and other white matter pathways in recovery of spontaneous speech. *Brain*. 1989;112 (Pt 1):1-38.

[33] Rioult-Pedotti MS, Friedman D, Hess G, Donoghue JP. Strengthening of horizontal cortical connections following skill learning. *Nat. Neurosci*. 1998;1(3):230-4.

[34] Liepert J, Bauder H, Wolfgang HR, Miltner WH, Taub E, Weiller C. Treatment-induced cortical reorganization after stroke in humans. *Stroke*. 2000;31(6):1210-6.

[35] Lascano AM, Grouiller F, Genetti M, Spinelli L, Seeck M, Schaller K, et al. Surgically relevant localization of the central sulcus with high-density somatosensory-evoked potentials compared with functional magnetic resonance imaging. *Neurosurgery*. 2014;74(5):517-26.

[36] Hayashi Y, Nakada M, Kinoshita M, Hamada J. Functional reorganization in the patient with progressing glioma of the pure primary motor cortex: a case report with special reference to the topographic central sulcus defined by somatosensory-evoked potential. *World Neurosurg*. 2014;82(3-4):536 e1-4.

[37] Robles SG, Gatignol P, Lehericy S, Duffau H. Long-term brain plasticity allowing a multistage surgical approach to World Health Organization Grade II gliomas in eloquent areas. *J. Neurosurg*. 2008;109(4):615-24.

[38] Bello L, Gambini A, Castellano A, Carrabba G, Acerbi F, Fava E, et al. Motor and language DTI Fiber Tracking combined with intraoperative subcortical mapping for surgical removal of gliomas. *Neuroimage*. 2008;39(1):369-82.

[39] Roux FE, Boulanouar K, Lotterie JA, Mejdoubi M, LeSage JP, Berry I. Language functional magnetic resonance imaging in preoperative assessment of language areas: correlation with direct cortical stimulation. *Neurosurgery*. 2003;52(6):1335-45; discussion 45-7.

[40] FitzGerald DB, Cosgrove GR, Ronner S, Jiang H, Buchbinder BR, Belliveau JW, et al. Location of language in the cortex: a comparison between functional MR imaging and electrocortical stimulation. *AJNR Am. J. Neuroradiol*. 1997;18(8):1529-39.

[41] Gilbert MR. Minding the Ps and Qs: perseverance and quality studies lead to major advances in patients with anaplastic oligodendroglioma. *J. Clin. Oncol*. 2013;31(3):299-300.

[42] Kang HC, Kim IH, Eom KY, Kim JH, Jung HW. The role of radiotherapy in the treatment of newly diagnosed supratentorial low-grade oligodendrogliomas: comparative analysis with immediate radiotherapy versus surgery alone. *Cancer Res. Treat*. 2009;41(3):132-7.

[43] Cairncross G, Berkey B, Shaw E, Jenkins R, Scheithauer B, Brachman D, et al. Phase III trial of chemotherapy plus radiotherapy compared with radiotherapy alone for pure and mixed anaplastic oligodendroglioma: Intergroup Radiation Therapy Oncology Group Trial 9402. *J. Clin. Oncol*. 2006;24(18):2707-14.

[44] Talagas M, Marcorelles P, Uguen A, Redon S, Quintin-Roue I, Costa S, et al. Identification of a novel population in high-grade oligodendroglial tumors not deleted on 1p/19q using array CGH. *J. Neurooncol*. 2012;109(2):405-13.

[45] Quon H, Hasbini A, Cougnard J, Djafari L, Lacroix C, Abdulkarim B. Assessment of tumor angiogenesis as a prognostic factor of survival in patients with oligodendroglioma. *J. Neurooncol*. 2010;96(2):277-85.

[46] Schiffer D, Dutto A, Cavalla P, Bosone I, Chio A, Villani R, et al. Prognostic factors in oligodendroglioma. *Can. J. Neurol. Sci*. 1997;24(4):313-9.

INDEX

#

A

B

C

D

E

F

G

H

I

K

L

M

N

O

P

T

U

V

W

Y